PSYCHIATRY: EDUCATION AND IMAGE

Psychiatry: Education and Image

Edited by

GENE USDIN, M.D.

Clinical Professor of Psychiatry
Louisiana State University School of Medicine

BRUNNER/MAZEL, *PUBLISHERS* • NEW YORK

Published by Brunner/Mazel, Inc.
64 University Place, New York, N. Y. 10003

Library of Congress Catalogue Card No. 73-85911

SBN 87630-078-6

MANUFACTURED IN THE UNITED STATES OF AMERICA

American College of Psychiatrists

OFFICERS

Benjamin Balser, M.D., *President*

Melvin Sabshin, M.D.
President-Elect

Hamilton Ford, M.D.
First Vice-President

Hayden H. Donahue, M.D.
Second Vice-President

Peter A. Martin, M.D.
Secretary-General

Charles E. Smith, M.D.
Treasurer

John D. Trawick, Jr., M.D.
Archivist-Historian

Program Committee for 1973 Annual Meeting

Gene Usdin, M.D., *Chairman*

Norman Q. Brill, M.D.
Duncan Burford, M.D.
Robert Gibson, M.D.
Donald Greaves, M.D.
Harold Hiatt, M.D.
S. Mouchly Small, M.D.
Perry C. Talkington, M.D.
Robert Williams, M.D.

Publications Committee for 1973 Annual Meeting

Gene Usdin, M.D., *Chairman*
Charles K. Hofling, M.D., *Vice-Chairman*

Earl Brown, M.D.
Paul Jay Fink, M.D.
Henry P. Laughlin, M.D.
John C. Nemiah, M.D.
Melvin Sabshin, M.D.
Harold Visotsky, M.D.

Contributors

JOHN J. SCHWAB, M.D.
Professor of Psychiatry, College of Medicine, University of Florida

RUBY B. SCHWAB

JUDD MARMOR, M.D.
Franz Alexander Professor of Psychiatry, University of Southern California School of Medicine

ROBERT L. ROBINSON
Director of Public Affairs, American Psychiatric Association

HENRY H. WORK, M.D.
Chief, Professional Services, American Psychiatric Association

JOHN P. HUBBARD, M.D.
President, National Board of Medical Examiners

BRYCE TEMPLETON, M.D.
Co-Director, Division of Graduate Medical Evaluation, National Board of Medical Examiners

THE REVEREND JOHN S. JENKINS
Rector, Trinity Episcopal Church, New Orleans

PETER A. MARTIN, M.D.
Clinical Professor of Psychiatry, University of Michigan and Wayne State University Medical School; Lecturer, Michigan Psychoanalytic Institute

HAROLD I. LIEF, M.D.
Professor of Psychiatry, Director, Division of Family Study; Director, Marriage Council of Philadelphia; Director, Center for the Study of Sex Education in Medicine

BERNARD C. HOLLAND, M.D.
Professor and Chairman, Department of Psychiatry, Emory University School of Medicine

ROBERT J. STOLLER, M.D.
Professor of Psychiatry, UCLA School of Medicine

PETER F. REGAN, M.D.
Professor of Psychiatry and Buswell Fellow, State University of New York at Buffalo, School of Medicine

S. MOUCHLY SMALL, M.D.
Professor and Chairman, Department of Psychiatry, and Buswell Fellow, State University of New York at Buffalo, School of Medicine

Contents

Introduction

Although the element of change is characteristic of the dynamics associated with all societal institutions, it frequently constitutes a serious threat to those members of a group who prefer reliance on the sterile cocoon of what they consider to be "time-tested knowledge" to the heady atmosphere of new and improved methods, expanded data, and fuller competence in the delivery of service.

Psychiatry: Education and Image holds the mirror before each reader who is engaged in the practice of psychiatry and its ancillary areas. It seeks to eliminate the distortions of self-evaluation and to focus—with a high degree of clarity—on the image the profession presents to the community at large. The authors of the nine presentations join in sounding a clarion call, summoning the practitioner to a recognition of worthwhile change achieved, change in progress, and change anticipated within the profession. They seek to admonish him to "put on the new man" lest scientific progress and changing needs render his once acceptable level of competence an anachronism. They seem to say that the winds of change are whispering, ever so gently, ever so persistently, ever so convincingly to those who are willing to listen and to move with the times. And they warn that failure to heed the gentle wind will find psychiatry unprepared for those coming forces—of hurricane proportion—which stand ready to impose change from without.

The parameters offered by the authors have the capacity to generate strong negative feelings and insecurity among those who find change threatening. However, these colleagues write with a precision, candor, and directness which should earn the respect of even those readers who may be inclined to disagree with the premises upon which the positions of the authors are based.

The contents of this volume cover a wide variety of subjects. The authors address past and current criticisms of psychiatry, suggest new approaches to the preparatory education of those seeking to enter the profession, and outline the continuing educational programs established practitioners will be expected to undertake in order to demonstrate periodically their competence to remain in practice. They write of systems of delivery of care and suggest how improvements may be introduced. They direct attention to a variety of new psychotherapeutic techniques, and even review the updated position of some clergymen. Distressing as it may appear, there is a suggestion that still a new category of professional is required in order that child advocacy may become a viable component of the total mental health effort, and strong arguments are presented for a more effective approach to the unmet demand for better marital counseling. The epidemiology of mental illness is reviewed, and the image and role of the psychiatrist are critically re-examined. All in all, the authors have joined in presenting a well developed, well integrated approach to an "in the family" evaluative inventory of psychiatry today. Hopefully, the signals which they fly from the masthead of their chapters will be clearly and appreciatively read by all to whom this book comes.

The initial chapter in this volume, written by the American Psychiatric Association's Director of Public Affairs, Robert L. Robinson, is a candid appraisal of our current image. He maintains that the present epidemic of criticism is possibly the worst we have experienced. Certainly the limelight into which psychiatry has been thrust and has thrust itself provides an appealing target, especially with the increasing expansion of the media coverage. Robinson reviews the major critiques of psychiatry, beginning with S. Weir Mitchell's address in 1893 to the mental hospital superintendents, and concluding with the far ranging onslaught of Thomas Szasz, who finds as his occasional bedfellows such diverse groups as the Birchites, the scientologists, some solid organicists, and many civil libertarians. No serious thinker can deny that Szasz's writings have been of some value; he has jolted the profession into a study of many practices—but he has also provided fuel to anti-mental health forces and other destructive groups. He has caused many to turn away from or be denied the benefits of psychiatric care when appropriate and needed. It is somewhat ironical that Szasz has become the most widely known psychiatrist in legal and psychological circles. Robinson also discusses the important criticisms of Alan Gregg, Desmond Curran, Percival Bailey and Roy Grinker, Sr. He poses problems with respect to our image, cites realistic dangers, offers specific suggestions, and concludes with a hopeful note contingent upon increased involvement of psychiatrists in our national organization. He expresses confidence that, now that the crisis has arisen, the leaders of American psychiatry will guide us effectively in confronting the issues and improving our training, services and image.

Henry H. Work, Chief of Professional Services of the American Psychiatric Association, presents a strong indictment of the failure to provide an adequate system of child care and emphasizes the need for an aggressive spokesman to procure such appropriately. He examines the legal, medical and educational models of advocacy for children which have begun to appear on both the national and local scenes and finds them discouraging and deficient. Work suggests the desirability of a new type of sub-professional to promote more effectively the care of children. This could be disturbing to many of those who are distressed by the proliferation of the conglomerate of sub-professionals currently participating in the delivery of care—often without adequate training. As an illustration of the potential difficulties of the new child-caring profession, he cited the work of the Parent-Child Centers established in recent years by the federal government. The question of inadequate training of individuals concerned with the delicate problem of child-rearing is discussed as part of a problem of the new professionals generally. Aggressive advocacy is needed but it must be continually mandated and supervised from the top.

There may be an implicit question in the title of Reverend Jenkins' chapter and his essay. What are the changing roles of the psychiatrists and clergy? May psychiatrists be becoming more superego directed, while the cleric in his ministering is becoming more receptive to the id needs of his parishioners? Are we witnessing, to some extent, a role reversal?

It is only within the past two or three centuries that the word "conscience" has lost its primary meaning of "knowing" and has taken on the more restricted connotation of "knowledge of good and bad," surrendering to a term of more recent coinage, "consciousness," its original, more general referent. Jenkins notes that, in the analytic model, the "superego" is roughly equatable with "conscience," and that the superego is only a portion of the totality of the psyche, which is conceived of as being comprised of ego, superego and id. Ideally, the analyst pays attention to all three aspects of his patients' psychic lives. In practice, there is a tendency for interest in one to dominate the others. Freud's early focus on id phenomena (viewed as libidinal in his earlier topographic model) is well known. In the late twenties and early thirties interest in the superego held the stage, especially in the work of Alexander and those influenced by him. Since the time of Hartmann, the ego and ego analysis have been the primary concern of clinicians and theoreticians alike.

The spotlight of consciousness can rarely illuminate more than one or two concepts at a time, and it is perhaps not surprising, therefore, that analysts have tended to single out and emphasize one psychic function at the expense of another. As Jenkins so cogently demonstrates, the same narrowness of vision afflicts those other explorers of the human soul, the priests and ministers of Christianity. They limit their vision, he argues, at the expense of a viable religion. Is there a lesson to be learned here by the psychiatrist, with his contemporary, perhaps overly-constricted focus on ego psychology to the virtual exclusion of other aspects of the psyche? As we search for our image as psychiatrists and our goals as medical healers of the emotionally ill, we would do well to read and ponder this cleric's presentation to ascertain the extent of its application to ourselves.

The Schwabs outline the realistic conceptual and methodological problems in studying the epidemiology of mental illness, emphasizing among other things the *sine qua non* of being aware of a particular society's values. They review some of the historic endeavors to meet the conceptual and methodological problems and use these examples to illustrate difficulties confronting investigators today. They note the defining of a "case" as critical, discuss medical and social criteria which have been developed, and assess the various models which have been applied, starting with Graunt's epidemiologic study published in 1662. They point out the social importance of exclusion, society's apparent need to eliminate, extrude, or immure a certain segment of the population. Historically, Western society has used the *Narrenschiffen,* bonfires, and houses of confinement to achieve this end. Since the seventeenth century, the practice of shuttling the poor back and forth between the asylum and the alms house has been repeated innumerable times. The Schwabs maintain that much of the problem of poverty and mental illness may stem from society's values. They conclude with a brief discussion of the importance of recognizing that our ideologies and values are dominant influences, and they highlight the need for descriptive epidemiology based on a phenomenological approach, as well as the need for a humanistic orientation to provide meaning to the epidemiology of mental health and illness.

Marmor follows with a review of relatively recent psychotherapeutic techniques, especially noting those that have emerged in this country since World War II. Marmor has never hesitated to state his beliefs clearly and strongly, and his chapter is a striking example of this. He has always been a pragmatist, willing to give up earlier concepts when they no longer are tenable in the light of newer experiences or studies. He has annoyed those who are unwilling to venture forth from their shelter of long cherished beliefs which provide them with a special therapeutic armamentarium. His criticism of orthodox analytic dogmatists and his plea for the integration of behavioral therapy concepts and methods with those of dynamic psychotherapy are certain to arouse many readers. Likewise, his encouragement of group therapies as a highly effective measure for mobilizing behavioral change will challenge those who feel the dyadic relationship is the only one of lasting therapeutic value. His iconoclasm may further antagonize his colleagues when he anticipates the decreasing resistance by many psychoanalytically oriented psychiatrists to the adjunctive use of appropriate psychopharmacologic agents. It is obvious that the process of hardening, of increasing rigidity, has never influenced Marmor, who in this chapter admirably personifies the eclecticist with a wide range of observation and opinion.

The chapter by Hubbard and Templeton will generate anxieties in many psychiatrists, possibly in correlation to their age or years away from residency training and direct clinical experience. The authors raise a critical issue in suggesting that a significant number of leaders of American psychiatry, organizational or academic, are years removed from clinical experience and maintain their security and their potency through their leadership roles, well developed political acumen, or demonstrable administrative skills.

Hubbard and Templeton emphasize the imperative need for additional factual data to guide the specialty of psychiatry as it faces challenges arising from the educational system and from society. The trends in medical education, cited in their chapter, have already produced a tremendous impact on the education of younger psychiatrists. We are currently experiencing some of these effects, and we shall doubtlessly experience even more important effects as the concepts cited by Hubbard and Templeton materialize through further developmental processes.

Although the subject is anxiety-provoking, the end is not yet in sight and may be more benign than anticipated. Since pre-medical training is now to be the preparation for graduate medical education, the residency becomes the training ground for the practice of medicine. Hubbard and Templeton argue that the experience of the resident in psychiatry must be broadened and must move toward a more thorough integration with the practice of medicine. Contrary directions tend to particularize further the already fragmented management of patient care with resultant alienation of psychiatry from the mainstream of medical practice.

Hubbard and Templeton call for a more precise definition of the qualifications for the practice of psychiatry. They suggest that certification should be required even before licensure. A more precise definition of the qualifications of a psychiatrist is indeed sorely needed. However, it may be virtually impossible to obtain agreement among psychiatrists on such a definition. There is, consequently, a danger that the qualifications to practice psychiatry may be imposed by legislative fiat. Proof of continuing competence in psychiatry is even more difficult to define. Many of us shudder at the thought of any group, in or out of psychiatry, periodically assessing one's competence to continue practicing the art. However, it is felt that such assessment will ultimately be required. Therefore, we in psychiatry must establish suitable standards before they are imposed upon us by outside authority resulting in undue and unrealistic constraints on practitioners adequately resolving at least part of the current need.

There is an urgent need for the formulation of educational objectives, the development of self-instructional techniques, and establishment of evaluative standards by which student progress may be measured in our residency programs. Guidance in these areas should be sought from recognized specialists from outside psychiatry as well as from within. Hubbard and Templeton offer material for serious contemplation and lively discussion. But such a discussion should lead to undertaking a hard look at what we expect psychiatry to be. If indeed we are faced with the task of initiating educational change, it should be presumed that we have clarified to our satisfaction the role the practitioner is called upon to play. Have members of our profession reached that position? Psychiatry would be hard put to accommodate credentials criteria in the manner of secondary and collegiate education. The secondary school teacher is a generalist with specialist training, equipped to function in a highly structured setting which has the mandate to develop the total child. The college instructor is much more frequently found to be highly specialized, single purposed, and not competent outside his own discipline and its literature. The secondary educator is more properly a generalist who can—without too great an expenditure of effort—move to cope with subject matter in courses other than the one he generally teaches.

Martin and Lief, mature, experienced clinicians long involved with medical education, indict psychiatric training which exhibits undue resistance to change. They explore the factors generally playing a part in the resistance to change in all psychiatric training by utilizing the example of resistance to the introduction of marital therapy courses into residency training programs. They suggest that the major portion of the resistance is attributable to fears of investigations of newer forms of treatment. Such avoidance results in a dearth of teachers skilled in these new areas. They document the importance of marital therapy, while affirming that minimal inroads have been made in introducing marital therapy training in the basic medical curriculum, but recognize that the same phenomena are present with innovation in other areas of the curriculum.

In a way, they are maintaining that the potency of psychiatric leaders is often threatened when their present model of technique is questioned and newer concepts have to be learned. It is as if the leaders have achieved eminence in their professions by their own concepts. Many are no longer engaged in direct patient care, research studies, or any semblance of clinical involvement. It is as if, having achieved their autonomy, they may experience a type of identity crisis or identity confusion through the infiltration of newer concepts which they find difficult to integrate.

Holland and Stoller point out that psychiatrists cannot be spared the turmoil that the evolution of our profession has produced. They draw attention to the blurred image of psychiatry and psychotherapy and raise the question of what is essential in psychiatric training. The authors note the different roles of individual psychiatrists and question the future of psychiatry as a profession. They review the risks to which psychiatry is being subjected, and ask whether it serves the patient. They feel our optimism far exceeds our capacity and suggest that we have identified and publicized a need we cannot resolve. They indicate that too often our methods appear uncertain, incomplete or insufficient. They state that we frequently react as though we have been misunderstood and harshly judged, and that we fail to appreciate fully the contribution we have made toward developing the predicament in which we find ourselves. They also give recognition to rising hopes in the midst of social inequity and take measure of our inability to meet those hopes for any wide proportion of the community, despite publicized treatment advances and improvement in our image as healers.

There can be little question that we have used the medical model as a sword and a shield and that this model is inappropriate for managing much of mankind's pain and unhappiness. Others, without a medical degree, have proven their capacity to treat. The authors' conclusion envisions the professional psychiatrist as a biologist of the human animal, broadly trained in the many perspectives of human psychology, skillful in diagnosis, prepared to select and prescribe optimally suited treatments, and trustworthy in the sense of responsibility comparable to that traditional for the physician. These qualifications, Doctors Holland and Stoller feel, identify the psychiatrist and separate him from the other mental health therapists.

The concluding portion of this volume by Regan and Small outlines the dilemma associated with predicting the future of medical education and implicitly points out the added difficulties which relate to psychiatry. There is a strong plea for extensive continuing education and lifelong habits of learning consonant with the increasing requirements for services. There is a demand that services be distributed more equitably and under continual surveillance. There has been an explosive increase of psychiatrists in the United States, and there are now more than 125 health professions and occupations, with increasing governmental involvement. The authors express concern about the collision course, intimately tied to the ever mounting public demand for service. They offer a partial solution in an abbreviated formal medical education with earlier specialization encouraged by multiple-track systems. They note that basic research may decrease and that imposition of controls may become more prominent. They view psychiatric education as a lifelong continuum and argue that major changes will have to be made in psychiatric training programs. Their outline is concise and specific regarding basic medical, as well as basic psychiatric and advanced psychiatric, education. They note the need for elective psychiatric courses, together with systematic continuing education. They voice an imperative need for the eclectic psychiatrist with an educational flexibility far beyond what most have considered. In spite of the complexity, there is a plea for more individualization in the training and continuing education of today's and tomorrow's psychiatrists.

What becomes apparent throughout this volume is that the psychiatrist will never have his old world again, and that the rapid explosion of knowledge will create stress and responsibilities such as psychiatrists of twenty years ago never contemplated. Psychiatrists, like others (maybe even more so), are prone to get on a bandwagon. The track system with accelerated training and diminished basic medical knowledge is currently the vogue for many. Many able psychiatric leaders question this development and deplore the decreased general medical training of the psychiatrist, as well as of other specialists. The battle lines have already been drawn regarding our moving away from the medical model to a behavioral type of team model. Psychiatrists, as well as other physicians, are personally threatened by advances which they nonetheless recognize as advisable for a better healing profession. Peer review and relicensure appear to be imminent. Both of these require extra time and raise additional threats.

As the presentations of these authors unfold multiple and varied innovations which advance upon the citadel of a traditional psychiatry, let us reflect on the preamble of this introduction. There we suggested that change was characteristic of societal institutions, and that change can be threatening. But change is characteristic of all viable institutions, and the absence of change is still more threatening, for it signifies death. At the same time, inevitability of change need not be feared, since society can exercise sufficient control over the character of the change as well as the rate at which it proceeds. Psychiatry has the opportunity to come of age and, as a cardinal component of the medical profession, to establish itself as a major contributor to the betterment of mankind.

This publication by the American College of Psychiatrists of the papers presented at its January, 1973 teaching symposium discusses these timely issues and presents educational guidelines and models for the psychiatry of tomorrow. The challenge implicit in our methods of education will substantially affect our image, both within and out of the medical profession. Only to the extent that we meet this challenge will psychiatry advance in strength and effectiveness.

GENE USDIN, M.D.

PSYCHIATRY: EDUCATION AND IMAGE

1.

Criticisms of Psychiatry

ROBERT L. ROBINSON

For those of us who are closely involved in psychiatry, it is important to consider criticisms from within as well as from without. Self-scrutiny becomes especially important when there is a period of rapid change and innovation. Certainly these past two decades have witnessed dramatic changes insofar as the theory and practice of psychiatry are concerned. The boundaries of psychodynamic applications have been extended into wide parameters while critics of psychiatry decry its value in any way.

In 1963 Miller and Halleck (1) outlined an impressive array of major patterns of criticism of psychiatry, most of which will be touched on in this presentation, but with considerable embellishment and expansion. They made clear their concern that psychiatry appeared to be at once the most prestigious and the most criticized profession on the American scene. They noted what they deemed a tendency on the part of the profession not to listen carefully to the content of criticism, and to refuse or resist the benefits of it, much less to do anything about it. They suggested that among psychodynamicists there is a disposition to focus on motivations for the criticism rather than with the criticism itself. After their extensive review of the literature, Miller and Halleck ventured that it is just possible the assumptions that psychiatry is here to stay, that it is essentially solidly based, that its hypotheses, if not always proven, are at least viable, and that it is a widely accepted profession, might prove untenable.

Since 1963 criticisms of psychiatry have become even more widespread and their scope more inclusive.

It seems sensible to begin by noting Webster's Third International Dictionary gives two main meanings to the term "criticism." One is simply "faultfinding, disapproval, or objection." The other is "the art of evaluating or analyzing with knowledge and propriety... as moral values or the soundness of scientific hypotheses and procedures."

The category of "faultfinding, disapproval, or objection" encompasses what may loosely be called the "anti-psychiatry" movement of today—the kinds of criticisms levelled by the Birchites, the Scientologists, the various liberationist groups, the political radicals, and so on. We cannot afford to ignore them, nor shall we.

But the faultfinding criticism of our times seems to derive its heart's blood from the epochal evaluative criticisms that have arisen from within our own ranks and from disciplines very close to us. By "epochal" I mean criticisms of historical significance that have captured the imagination at the time they have appeared and have remained to guide us or haunt us since. I shall attempt brief summaries and interpretations, and some interpolation, of five of these, namely by Drs. S. Weir Mitchell, Alan Gregg, Desmond Curran, Percival Bailey, and Roy M. Grinker, Sr. To these I shall add a sixth, Dr. Thomas Szasz, in a special context.

Let me dwell briefly on Mitchell's stirring address to the mental hospital superintendents in 1893 (2) when he admonished them: "Your hospitals are not our hospitals; your ways are not our ways. You live out of range of critical shot; you are not preceded and followed in your ward work by clever rivals, or watched by able residents fresh with learning from the school." He castigated them for cultivating the notion that they, as medical superintendents, were also qualified as caterers, farmers, stewards, treasurers, business managers, and physicians. He asked them to "urge in every report the stupidity of this." In sum, he told them their hospitals were no damned good, that they were incompetent to run them, that they were poor physicians, and worse scientists, that they had isolated themselves from criticism that could lead to improvement, and that they had better change their ways. And he went so far as to say explicitly how they could go about setting up and operating decent hospitals for their charges if they but would.

Today one cannot dismiss Mitchell as a curiosity of history. Can one imagine that this lively mind would be much more pleased today than he was then with the status of our public mental hospitals? Certainly he would find some improvements, and he would say so. But what would he say of Willowbrook, of Bryce Hospital, of Atascadero? What would be his response to the charges of contemporary civil libertarians that our hospitals are "worse than prisons"; that many of their physicians are inadequately trained foreigners who do not even speak the language; that the involuntary patient is, in effect, a "prisoner of psychiatry?" What would Mitchell's stance be toward the judicial doctrine of "right to treatment?" It seems safe to guess he would have no small empathy with, and would provide authoritative grist for, certain elements of the anti-psychiatry movement today. And so it was that this epochal critic helped set afoot a whole pattern of criticism remaining very much with us.

Fifty years later, in 1944, on the occasion of the Centenary meeting of the American Psychiatric Association in Philadelphia, the great Alan Gregg (3), always a firm friend and an equally severe critic of psychiatry, proved somewhat kinder in his approach but no less incisive than Dr. Mitchell. At the time, psychiatrists had begun to move out of the asylums and into private practice, general hospitals and clinics. As though to ameliorate his criticisms, Dr. Gregg pinpointed three of the profession's heritages from which spring so many of its difficulties: the horror that mental disease has always inspired; the manifold and subtle ways in which psychiatric symptoms impinge adversely on human relations; and man's tendency to separate the spirit and the body, the psyche and the soma. He noted that no other profession has had to rescue its patients from persecution, or live with them in isolation, or restore their capacities only to return them to a hostile and suspicious environment. But among his most telling criticisms were these: ** The profession, by experience and status, is but ill prepared to accept criticism, and the task of the critic becomes unanimously resisted and as futile as it is invidious. ** Neither in quantity nor quality has psychiatry drawn from the medical schools the students appropriate to the nature and urgency of its need. ** As a natural consequence of their isolation, psychiatrists speak a dialect, a special lingo that produces more resentment than comprehension or interest on the part of their medical brethren, and so defeat the very object of language, which is the communciation of ideas. ** They distrust outsiders, and their petty loyalties often appear as the signature of the specialty. And finally, he concluded, "you are inarticulate." He did not blame the profession for its exasperation at being ignored... "but I tell you," he said, "that you and your millions of charges deserve better champions and more articulate spokesmen than have arisen from your ranks. . . . Must you forever rely on outsiders to tell the laity your overwhelming truths?"

It is relevant that he was nonetheless sanguine about the future of the field, venturing that psychiatry would find applications far beyond its hospitals and offices—applications in the human relations of normal people, in politics, national and international affairs, between races, in government, in family life, and in education. In short, he said, psychiatry would be concerned with "optimal performance of human beings as civilized creatures."

All in all, and curiously, Dr. Gregg's criticisms seem a little more dated today than Dr. Mitchell's. Perhaps we have in some measure learned better how to contend with criticism if for no other reason than that there has been so much of it. We have certainly made great strides in carving out a place for psychiatry in medical education, and psychiatry apparently is drawing off its full share of the bright young medical students of our time. Perhaps our lingo has not improved greatly, but certainly it has at least become more widely understood and some of it has been incorporated into the household vernacular of our times, e.g. "oedipal problems," "sibling rivalry," "paranoid personality," "unconscious wish," etc. But our progress has been less than impressive with regard to what I consider his most salient criticism: our willingness to allow outsiders to expound our "overwhelming truths" and to defend the millions in our charge while we remain relatively silent and inarticulate. Collectively, we do not speak with a strong voice; we remain a babel of many voices.

When Dr. Gregg spoke of the extension of psychiatry into many fields beyond the office and the hospital, he articulated a proposition that led straight to a critical response by another epochal critic, Dr. Desmond Curran, a British colleague (4). Dr. Curran's main criticism was an attack on the global proclivities of psychiatry, and he took as his point of departure the World Health Organization's definition of "health" as "a state of complete physical, mental, and social well being and not merely the absence of disease or infirmity." Psychiatry in general was pleased at the time, but Dr. Curran was alarmed.

He pointed to the doctor's dilemma that when he can find no physical pathological lesions in a complaining patient, then he must either conclude there is nothing wrong, which is clearly untenable, or he must search for explanations to cover an infinite variety of maladjustments. The problem is where to call his search to a halt. He said the World Health Organization definition could only be interpreted as saying to all people of the world: "If you're not healthy, then you are sick and since nobody is ever in a state of complete physical, mental, and social well being, then everybody is sick."

Obviously the definition provided an ideal platform to expand the medical, and particularly the psychiatric, roles *ad infinitum* along the lines Dr. Gregg had predicted. To sum it all up, Dr. Curran suggested, psychiatry perceived its responsibilities as falling short of nothing less than world reform. He questioned the wisdom of this, and made clear that the very notion was anathema to him and fraught with peril. "Is it really wise to look for new fields to conquer," he asked,"when so much needs to be done yet in the clinical field?" "I for one," he ventured, "have no yearning to run the world, and I can say with no false modesty I do not believe I could." He would convert psychiatry into a "limited liability company"—"a respectable company"—in which shareholders are not liable for more than they subscribe, a "large concern with big responsibilities and with a great future before it. The shareholders are quiet, diffident, modest, sober men who have a real pride in their business, but they are vexed when others undermine the reputation of the firm by using the name to float bogus companies, with grandiose prospectuses, backed up by balance sheets that do not add up to make sense."

Thus, by the early 1950s the basic thesis that psychiatry should limit its purview to that of the traditional physician and clinician, and the antithesis that it should expand to encompass the optimal performance of human beings as civilized creatures were well articulated, and this set afoot the dialectic that remains so far from resolution today. The debate has compounded in geometric proportions. Confusion is rampant within the profession and more so in the public's view. This is not to suggest that the profession has done anything wrong in stumbling, as it were, into this state of uncertainty, or this "identity crisis" if you will, but it does open the profession to a tornado of faultfinding criticism from those in the body politic who are predisposed to be contemptuous of it and are now the better positioned to point to our vagaries of purpose as justification enough for a speedy demise. And so they do.

Possibly the unkindest cut of all by way of epochal criticism of the profession was administered by Dr. Percival Bailey in 1956 at the Annual Meeting of the Association (5). Bitter in style, masterful in scholarly content (171 references), Dr. Bailey titled his address sardonically, "The Great Psychiatric Revolution." He reviewed the results of shock treatment, of psychosurgery, and of pharmacology and found them sorely wanting. But he reserved the hottest coals of criticism for psychoanalysis. He said, "In psychoanalysis I find no vision without which the people perish.... It has been banned in the Soviet Union because it treats society not as something which creates new forms of psychic life, but as a negative force which suppresses man's basic needs.... Its Master neglected and disdained women—half the human race—and admitted that he never understood them.... He completely ignored all spiritual values. He neglected the social nature of mankind. He developed no system of values. He neglected the fundamental human instinct of curiosity. . . . He overemphasized the unconscious. . . . He taught that civilization decreases happiness by increasing the feeling of guilt... (and) ...as Masserman puts it, he let his own formulations influence his therapy in the direction of pessimism, conservatism, and occasionally, even overt nihilism."

In sum, Dr. Bailey charged that "The Great Psychiatric Revolution" has solved few problems; the task of psychiatrists seemed to him to be "to get back into the asylums and laboratories which they are so proud to have left behind them and prove, by established criteria, that their concepts have scientific validity." He stated his own conviction that the problem of the psychoses would in time be solved by biochemists.

For seven years prior to Dr. Bailey's critique, the author had been building up the press relations of the Association. You may be sure that Dr. Bailey's remarks were manna from heaven to the reporters who attended the meeting where he made them. Unquestionably Dr. Bailey contributed enormously to receptivity of the public to the proposition which has been so prominently featured in the lay media in the past decade that psychoanalysis is either dying, or indeed is already dead.

Less than a decade later Dr. William Sargant (6) in a special supplement published by *Atlantic* magazine in July 1964 alleged that one had to be a psychoanalyst to hold high position in American psychiatry and implied that British psychiatry was superior because it labored under no such handicap. Sargant's criticism was scarcely an epochal one; rather it fell into the category of disapproving, faultfinding criticism. But we cannot deny the fact that many decision-makers in American society were moved by it. For example, in the October 1964 issue of *The Atlantic Monthly,* the eminent scientist Vannevar Bush wrote: "Sargant's assault on the psychoanalysts was needed and convincing. He certainly did not use the word 'racket' but he certainly implied it. A good job all around." And Walter Lippman, the dean of newspaper columnists, said of the special supplement: "It was a great public service."

To return to epochal criticisms, Dr. Roy Grinker, Sr. in 1964 (7) took note, with implicit disapproval, of the public image of psychiatrists as "magical helpers" who know the unknowable, who can interpret a glance, a gesture, a slipped word, or a phrase to mean so much. Often the psychiatrist is endowed with all of the powers of a supernatural father. The press prints our comments on all manner of problems of everyday life. But the other side of the coin is that to many sophisticates we are quacks, charlatans, and pretentious bores. As had Bailey, Dr. Grinker cited his disenchantment with psychoanalysis, which he found mired in a theoretical rut, vigilantly guarded by the orthodox.

He noted that the definition of psychiatry as the medical science of preventing and treating the mental disorders has somehow been grossly expanded, that the field now appears to encompass anything from biodynamics to philosophy, and truly rides madly in all directions. "Psychiatry," he said, "seems to suck in partial ideas as soon as they are announced as if it were a vacuum abhorring itself." "Have we nothing of our own?" he asked. He pleaded for a renewed dedication to the education of "disciplined investigators who are committed to rigorous testing and searching. They would not fear to discard what others swear is true and would maintain a healthy skepticism about accepting without reasonable proof what is enthusiastically touted because it is new." Dr. Grinker, certainly a friendly critic, maintained his hope that there may one day be a science of man to which psychiatry will contribute significantly.

In essence, Dr. Grinker appealed for us to avoid the persiflage and repair to a sounder scientific base. I doubt that he would feel the profession is riding in any fewer directions today than in 1964, or that his cautions had not fallen on deaf ears.

A final epochal criticism, of a quite different genre, one that has wreaked the most havoc with the profession in the past decade, has been that of Dr. Thomas Szasz (8,9,10,11).

His postulates are well known and need not be reviewed here. Dr. Szasz apparently envisages a continuing role for the profession of which he is a part; that is, he allows that anyone who wants to consult a psychiatrist should be able to and might even be comforted by doing so. But otherwise he disowns virtually in their entirety the foundations on which the profession so uneasily rests. He is not a very distant relative of a body of alienated extremists symbolized, for example, by one of our own, Dr. Paul Lowinger, a leader in APA's Radical Caucus, who tells us (12) that his first order of business is the destruction of the American Psychatric Association. Suffice it here that the impact of Szaszian thought on certain segments of the American intelligentsia, particularly the legal profession and civil libertarians, has been enormous—not to mention the ammunition he has provided to extremists of all hues, including Birchites and Scientologists. Within the narrow confines of this paper, the nature of that impact in high places will be merely suggested.

For example, last year Thomas L. Shaeffer (13), Dean and Professor of Law at Notre Dame Law School, addressing a session of the Catholic Hospital Association in Chicago, called upon the health professions "to empty every mental institution finally and completely, of every patient who wants to leave." He said, in so many words, if a kookie citizen wants to be a kook he has the right to be a kook and not be locked up. "I am asking you to open up mental treatment, put it on a free enterprise basis"—and this as a matter of fundamental constitutional right. As for the "dangerous" people, other institutions can take care of these. "The fact is that commitment to a mental institution is a life sentence to a place that is probably worse than prison." Thus Dean Shaeffer's reading of the gospel according to Thomas Szasz.

Indeed, it is fair to state that Dr. Szasz has inspired a whole new school of civil libertarians to launch a massive campaign against involuntary treatment for the mentally ill. A good example appears in a recent book by Bruce Ennis (14), a bright young lawyer, titled *Prisoners of Psychiatry,* with an Introduction by Dr. Szasz. It is based on his experiences with a special project he directed under the auspices of the New York Civil Liberties Union over the past three years. It is worth your attention. Mr. Ennis is not bitter against psychiatrists as individuals, but against the "system." In his view, psychiatry is no closer to understanding mental illness than it was decades ago. Hospital stays are shorter than then, but he says that is because the hospitals are admitting more and more persons who are only mildly disturbed. He asserts that our nomenclature remains ambiguous, meaning whatever the examiner wants it to mean; that the hospitals are filled with unlicensed foreign doctors; that the mental hospital system is governed not by laws, but by men who make their own laws; that medical terms are a disguise for social judgments; that psychiatrists are no good at predicting dangerous behavior, being wrong more often than they are right; that we tolerate all manner of vagueness in our mental hygiene laws that would not be tolerated in the criminal law. And in this vein Mr. Ennis purveys the Szaszian line.

The threads of Szaszian thought find their way into a legion of critical quarters today. Just in passing, we must take brief note of the "Nader Report" on the National Institute of Mental Health, and comunity mental health centers (15). Among other things the authors charge: The assumption that the community mental health centers must be inextricably linked to the psychiatric profession, and its medical orientation to the treatment of "diseases" has been the "albatross" of the centers program. Discontinue the use of medical model in all mental health facilities, they say. Plan now for the final demise of the state hospitals and pass laws inhibiting admissions to them. Confine the role of psychiatrists and physicians to treating definable medical problems. Convert the centers to human service agencies. Surely, the tenor of these recommendations reflects a strong admixture of the Szaszian approach to the field.

So much for six "epochal criticisms" of psychiatry. There are others which could be cited; but these will suffice. They have been reviewed at some length because they provide the basic authoritative themes that can be used by critics of all kinds.

Mix these ingredients, if you will, and what do we have? Take Mitchell's theme which intoned: You are not really doctors, you are something else; your ways are not our ways, and your public institutions are a disgrace. Combine with Bailey's disenchantment wtih psychiatry's treatment record and with psychoanalysis in particular. Then add Curran's charge that psychiatry seems bent on reforming the world without having the slightest competence to do so. Add Grinker's echo that we seem to ride madly in all directions. Slip in a fillip of Gregg that we are poor spokesmen either for ourselves or the millions of our charges. Top off the mixture with "Essence of Szasz" and we conjure a gooey concoction that the author, as Director of Public Affairs of the APA, has found neither palatable or simple to deal with.

Now let us depart from these epochal themes and from our own and closely related disciplines, and skirt quickly over the landscape of psychiatric criticism from other sources and in the various media.

Ponder for a moment the psychiatrist as pictured in the American novel and on the stage since World War I. Winnick spelled this out in 1963 (16) and Rogow, in some measure, brought it up to date in 1970 (17).

You may take the word of these scholars who have analyzed the characters of several dozen popular novels and plays that, with a very few exceptions, the fictional psychiatrist is evil, capable of indescribable outrage, a spoiled priest, cold and unfeeling, a blackmailer of patients, bizarre in behavior, despised by medical colleagues, a celebrity chaser, a seducer of young women, incompetent, lacking in common sense, a quack, a murderer, a sadist, comical, ridiculous, and reactionary—an anything but edifying picture.

Possibly in the case of the novelists and dramatists, the ugly treatment of the psychiatrist can, in large part, be explained by unconscious factors at work in the creative mind. But I call attention to the reality that much of the grist which goes into the making of their perverse and distorted characters derives from the artists' perceptions of the gooey concoction to which I have referred. Combined with their imagination, their desire to entertain, and to sell their books, the epochal criticisms and their derivatives assist these artists in conjuring all manner of horror stories in which the psychiatrist is the villain.

We come out a little better at the hands of cartoonists. Some are genuinely funny, gentle, and good humored. But all too many, as Dr. Henry Davidson has pointed out, feature the psychiatrist as a buffoon and fool wrapped up in trivia (18). Occasionally, a cartoon strikes one as ominous. For example, *Playboy* magazine (November 1972) recently portrayed a psychiatrist standing stark naked by his couch on which reclines an extremely well-stacked young lady. The caption read, "Today, Miss Simpson, in an effort to help you overcome your fear, I'm going to give you my shock treatment." This new license assumed by *Playboy* can only emanate from the rash of popular articles on "sex therapy" that have appeared in the popular media in the recent past, which, in turn, were inspired by "contributions to the literature," some of them respectable and some distinctly less so. The *Playboy* cartoon alerts one to an opinion spreading among a wide reading public that sexual relations between psychiatrist and patient are a common phenomenon.

It is not really relevant to discuss the treatment of psychiatry in the daily press here because news, by definition, is not criticism. That is not to say that news may not be a disaster, or that reporters do not sometimes bring to the style in which they present it a background of knowledge of the epochal criticisms. In this context, perhaps psychiatry's greatest news disaster of all time occurred in 1964 when some 10% of America's psychiatrists thought themselves competent to go on public record alleging that Barry Goldwater was psychologically unfit to be president of the United States. It seems doubtful that editorialists will ever allow psychiatry to forget this giant *gaffe*. From the standpoint of news coverage of the Goldwater affair, however, we were treated with remarkable charity. But that is a story in itself. As one who reviews thousands of news clippings covering the field, let me say categorically that we are treated decently by the press in the main.

Nor shall I attempt to analyze at any length the treatment of psychiatry in the most telling medium of all, television. It is common to feature psychiatrists on various kinds of television "talk shows" on such subjects as psychiatry in general, homosexuality, sexual freedom, bringing up children, women's liberation, and so on. It is rather rare, however, for the TV networks to feature psychiatrists or psychiatry, except incidentally, in purely entertainment productions or serials. In the few that I have seen, the image has been a benign one, albeit distorted and divorced from reality. I suspect that the networks do not think the public is quite ready for "hard core psychiatry." But they may come to it, and if they do, and if the opportunity can only be well managed—and that's a big *if*—psychiatry might do well to seize upon it to offset the distorted criticisms that continue to plague it.

The treatment of psychiatry in the media of the intelligentsia and the well-educated middle class is another thing again. I refer to such journals as *The Atlantic Monthly, Harper's, The New York Review, New Yorker, American Scholar, New Republic,* and the late lamented *Saturday Evening Post* and *Life Magazine.* It is largely through these media that the epochal criticisms are translated into meaningful language for the average intelligent citizens who are among the decision-makers in our society. It is incumbent on the profession to pay them great heed.

On rare occasions these criticisms have a direct impact on the profession. I think of the article by the distinguished journalist I. F. Stone, titled "Betrayal by Psychiatrists," which appeared in the influential *New York Review* about a year ago (February 1972). Mr. Stone hates all bureaucracies and their henchmen, and most especially the Soviet bureaucracy. He castigated the World Congress of Psychiatry, meeting in Mexico City in November 1971, for its failure to condemn the use of psychiatric institutions in the Soviet

Union for the suppression of dissenters; the fact that the APA had previously gone on record as condemning the practice "wherever it may occur" (without mentioning the Soviet Union) was, by no means, enough for Mr. Stone. His implication was that American psychiatrists were "moral cowards" pure and simple—poor spokesmen for their charges. Mr. Stone thoughtfully arranged for the *New York Review* to send to APA the documentation on which he based his article and demanded that we pass a judgment on it. *Mirabile dictu,* APA's trustees did appoint a Task Force to do just that! The Task Force found the documentation "impressive" and recommended that the World Psychiatric Association seek endorsement of APA's position on the matter by all of its member societies, including the Soviet psychiatric society.

Beyond that, the Task Force asked that its name be changed to "Ad Hoc Committee to Study Conflicts Inherent in the Therapeutic and Institutional Roles of Psychiatrists." The Trustees authorized this proposal, indicating the committee should look into such questions as whether the hospital superintendent, the military psychiatrist, the university health service psychiatrist, the industrial psychiatrist, and so on, are primarily serving the patients as healers of the sick, rather than serving the best interests of the institutions or the power structure from which they receive their salaries. You will readily sense what a thorny thicket we enter here, but at least psychiatry has shown the courage to grasp this nettle. Mr. Stone's criticism thus precipitated no small chain of events and a constructive response from the APA.

Another major critique of psychiatry was by Richard Lemon and appeared as a Special Supplement in the *Saturday*

Evening Post in August 1968 under the title, "Psychiatry, the Uncertain Science." This splendid and perceptive writer worked for three years in preparing the article. In effect, he brought up to date many of the epochal criticisms of psychiatry as of 1968.

Condensed and to some extent interpolated, some of his major points were:

> No one can say how well any of psychiatry's treatments work because there are no cures in the strict sense. Improvement and recovery are matters of subjective judgment.
>
> Psychiatrists as individuals are prickly and prone to disagreement.
>
> Psychiatrists do not even speak a common language. Leaders of various schools will refine lingos to a point where they baffle each other. As Karl Menninger says, "I can give you assurance that I cannot understand a good deal of what my colleagues are talking about."
>
> Instead of working to break down these differences, they are apt to be segregated from one another. They tend to work with others who share their own belief systems. As a result, psychiatry is like a large medieval country with a number of isolated fortresses in a climate that either is, or looks an awful lot like, war.
>
> The proliferation of experimental treatments of all kinds makes psychiatry an energetic profession. But so far it has had almost no success in converting that energy into a scientific body of information. As a result, psychiatrists are now in the unique position of helping the mentally ill in many ways and disagreeing among themselves about all of them.
>
> In sum, psychiatry today is a remarkable profession, racked by dissension, lacking established rules or prac-

> tices, unsure of its proper role in society, and flourishing anyway. It is not surprising that a profession in such shape should "turn off" many who come in contact with it. Some informed people consider it all bunk, and many more consider most of it bunk, as reflected in jokes about it. (*e.g.* "A psychiatrist is a Jewish doctor afraid of the sight of blood." Or, "Psychiatry is an unidentified technique applied to unspecified problems with unpredictable results.") But psychiatry doesn't deserve the scrap heap because the disagreements often appear more intense than they are. Many therapies have demonstrably worked for patients, and in the past decade psychiatry has accomplished more in the treatment of mental illness than ever before.

All psychiatrists will register a certain empathy for Mr. Lemon's points.

Departing from direct discussion of the media, we observe that psychiatry increasingly finds itself audited by comparable peers in other disciplines. This is especially true as the profession ventures far from its traditional medical pastures into other fields in the name of prevention. One small example will suffice to suggest others to you. When the Freud-Bullitt book on Woodrow Wilson was published, the distinguished historian, Barbara Tuchman, commented on it (19). She noted the book is full of factual error, obfuscations, misinterpretations, and all manner of biases. While Miss Tuchman believes the Freudian method can do much to shed light on the behavior of historical figures, she pleads, "Let it, for God's sake, be applied by a responsible historian."

Mention should be made of another dark cloud, already much bigger than a man's hand, that has been collecting on the horizon and now hovers immediately overhead. The responsible media are taking increasing note of it. This has to do with the charge that psychiatry operates two systems of care, one for the rich, one for the poor. Refer, for example, to a feature story by Michael T. Malloy in the *National Observer* for December 2, 1972, titled, "The Not Quite Doctors." He bases his article on a personal assessment of the situation in West Virginia's state hospital system where, he says, of 56 doctors employed to staff six state institutions, only five are licensed to practice medicine in the state. The author concluded that the institution of psychiatry will accommodate these unlicensed foreign medical school graduates because it helps at least to legitimize and sustain the medical model in these institutions, which is considered preferable to allowing, say, well-trained clinical psychologists, to function in their place. Such charges are, of course, commonplace in the literature of the civil libertarians and the followers of Szasz.

I have attempted to picture for you a limited, but nevertheless panoramic, view of patterns of criticism, the subtle forms they take, how they originate, how they proliferate, and the various impacts they have. Much has been left out—the complaints of your colleagues in other fields of medicine; the ravings and the rantings of the Birchites and the Scientologists; the sincere protestations of the women, the homosexuals, the minority groups, and your patients; the unkind cuts of the psychologists, sociologists, political scientists, and the judges and editorialists of all hues and colors. But all are the offspring of the patterns which have been traced. Nor have I attempted to answer the criticisms, or for the most part, suggested how they might be answered. But I am impelled to express a few personal opinions in concluding my remarks.

First, in spite of all, the author does not share Miller

and Halleck's concern, after their 1964 survey of the literature of criticism, that it may just possibly be that psychiatry is not a viable profession after all. The nub of the matter is that psychiatrists are physicians. I haven't the slightest doubt that they are going to remain physicians, and that the market for their services is here to stay. So be it.

But I do think psychiatry is in somewhat more serious trouble than it has yet realized, and that the trouble arises, importantly, out of the image of the profession that pervades the culture, an image derived largely from the patterns of criticism we have reviewed. Let me suggest an ominous note to illustrate cause for my concern.

Last October the *Wall Street Journal* (20) featured a lead article based on interviews with White House officials, including John Ehrlichman—who, as you know, was one of President Nixon's closest advisors. Mr. Ehrlichman made it "perfectly clear" to the reporter that the White House proposed to weed out "non-productive" programs. He said, "What we're talking about is a very hard-nosed analysis of cost effectiveness and the elimination of those programs that can't sustain the burden of proof. . . . I think a President with a substantial mandate, who feels the majority of people are behind him, will feel very comfortable in saying to a vested interest group, such as the social workers, 'Look, your social program of the 1960s isn't working, and we're going to dismantle it, so you'll just have to go out and find honest labor somewhere else.' " Mr. Ehrlichman went on to remark that "there are a lot of parasites sucking the fiscal blood."

Mr. Ehrlichman would not allow himself to be quoted on which parasites he had in mind, but the reporter left no doubt he had mentioned such agencies as OEO, HEW, and the National Institute of Mental Health. We know

now Mr. Ehrlichman was not kidding, for we have the Administration's proposed budget for fiscal 1974. Psychiatry has come upon dark days *vis-a-vis* the executive branch of government, which clearly regards its cost-effectiveness performance as considerably below par. The climate of accommodation we enjoyed so long has chilled to an unpleasant degree.

It is predictable that psychiatry will continue to suffer the outrage of critics in increasing degree until some substantial correction occurs between the disparity it offers in its treatment of the affluent and the poor. The profession is groping for answers—answers hopefully to be found in a gestalt that encompasses psychiatry in national health insurance, in community mental health centers, in health maintenance organizations, in the expansion of general hospital psychiatry, and so on. But the profession's mills sometimes grind exceedingly slow.

There is the problem of whether to straddle the fence of the medical and other models, or to jump to one side or the other. In the foreseeable future we cannot avoid straddling that fence. But it seems probable that psychiatry's crotch will endure many sharp pains as it veers first to this side, then to the other, in an effort to keep its balance. Perhaps the best solution lies in lowering the fence.

The venture into the human services area is, of course, related to charges of the profession's "globality" and the dangers inherent in that. I cannot resist quoting a comment by another kindly, but extremely incisive, critic of the profession and an ardent devotee of the medical model, Dr. Humphrey Osmond (21). Taking umbrage at the rhetoric of radical critics of the medical specialty of psychiatry he says:

> It is not psychiatry which is a fraud, but its pretensions as a panacea for every conceivable social and political ailment of our own and other times. So much of our energy has been dissipated by pretending that we have much competence in that vast miasmic swamp called mental health, which includes all our patients (a big enough helping for even the greatest gourmand), but also [includes] politics, foreign affairs, industrial relations, and much else.... We have plenty of patients. I wonder what the radicals will do with them while these grand plans and schemes are developing?

I am reasonably confident, however, that nature will, in the long run, provide adequate checks on hasty and excessive forays into fields relatively foreign to the psychiatrist. Nor do I think there should be an arbitrary intervention to prevent these forays. But they will bring trouble, for sure. Many chickens will come home to roost, and when they do, some of our very good people, unfortunately, are going to find themselves standing under their perch.

Finally, I do agree with Miller and Halleck that the profession as a whole does not adequately absorb, and therefore benefit from, the criticisms that attend it. Indeed, one cannot but suspect that great numbers of psychiatrists are not even aware of them. Those who are tend to resist the criticisms, to cast them aside as brickbats from the hostile, and sometimes to deny them altogether. That such response is not conducive to healthy maturation is obvious.

The situation is serious. It would be useful for the American Psychiatric Association to establish a commission of its best minds to make an ongoing study of criticisms of psychiatry, with the mission of analyzing and sorting out those of substance and conveying their essence to the profession at large, of rebutting some that deserve rebutting, and of recommending action programs in response to those that are on target. The author, for one, would find great comfort in the thoughtful and authoritative support of such a group in his own attempts to facilitate psychiatry's determination to do something for mankind.

REFERENCES

1. Miller, Milton and Halleck, Seymour: The Critics of Psychiatry: A Review of Contemporary Critical Attitudes. *Amer. J. Psychiat.,* vol. 119, No. 8, February, 1963.
2. Mitchell, S. Weir: Address to the 50th Annual Meeting, American Medico-Psychological Association, Philadelphia, 1893. *Translations of the AMPA,* vol. I, 1894, p. 101.
3. Gregg, Alan: A Critique of Psychiatry, Centenary Meeting of APA, Philadelphia, 1944. *Amer. J. Psychiat.,* vol. 101, Book I, p. 285.
4. Curran, Desmond, Psychiatry Limited. Presidential Address, Section on Psychiatry, Royal Society of Medicine, October 1951, *J. Ment. Science,* July, 1952.
5. Bailey, Percival: The Great Psychiatric Revolution. Academic Lecture, 112th Annual Meeting, APA, Chicago, 1956. *Amer. J. Psychiat.,* vol. 113, p. 387.
6. Sargant, William: Psychiatric Treatment: Here and in England. *The Atlantic Monthly,* July, 1964. (Part of Special Supplement on "Disturbed Americans.")
7. Grinker, Roy M.: Psychiatry Rides Madly in All Directions. *Arch. Gen. Psychiat.,* vol. 10, March 1964, p. 228.
8. Szasz, Thomas: *The Myth of Mental Illness.* New York: Hoeber-Harper, 1961.
9. Szasz, Thomas: *Ethics of Psychoanalysis.* New York: Basic Books, 1965.
10. Szasz, Thomas: *Law, Liberty and Psychiatry.* New York: Macmillan, 1963.
11. Szasz, Thomas: *Psychiatric Justice.* New York: Macmillan, 1965.
12. Lowinger, Paul: *Canadian Psychiatric Association Journal* (SS-II) 1972, p. 195.
13. Schaeffer, Thomas L.: A Lawyer's Plea: Open Mental Hospital Doors. Address to Catholic Hospital Assoc., Chicago, 1972. Reprinted in *National Observer,* Dec. 9, 1972.
14. Ennis, Bruce J.: *Prisoners of Psychiatry.* New York: Harcourt Brace, 1972.

15. Chu, Franklin and Trotter, Charlotte: *The Mental Health Complex, Community Mental Health Centers* (Part I), Task Force Report on the National Institute of Mental Health. Center for the Study of Responsive Law, Washington, D. C., 1972 (Mimeo).
16. Winnick, Charles: The Psychiatrist in Fiction. *J. Nerv. and Ment. Disease,* vol. 136, 1963, p. 43.
17. Rogow, Arnold: *The Psychiatrists.* New York: G. P. Putnam & Sons, 1970.
18. Davidson, Henry A.: The Image of the Psychiatrist. *Am. J. Psychiatry,* vol. 121, Oct. 1964, pp. 329-334.
19. Tuchman, Barbara: Comment in *The Atlantic Monthly,* Feb. 1967 on *Woodrow Wilson: Twenty-Eighth President of the United States—A Psychological Study.* New York: Houghton Mifflin, 1967.
20. Gannon, James P.: If President Wins Again the Nation May Have a Do Less Government. *Wall Street Journal,* Oct. 18, 1972, p. 1.
21. Osmond, Humphrey: Personal communication, Dec. 12, 1972.

2.

Advocacy for Children, 1973 "Need or Hope?"

HENRY H. WORK, M.D.

When the word "advocacy" first became current following the 1970 report of the Joint Commission on Mental Health of Children, it expressed a very real feeling that the children of the United States, despite all of the attention given them during this century, had been shortchanged. Numerous services, ostensibly designed to assist children in trouble as well as those making inadequate progress in the world, have been elaborated since the early days of the twentieth century. In spite of these, there appeared to be evidence that the services were poorly organized, that they failed to assist the very children for whom they were designed, and that there continued to be considerable antagonism to children as evidenced by the fact that many of the services appeared to be coercive in nature.

Since the organization of services for children has primarily been the responsibility of child psychiatrists, the image of this group of the profession has been somewhat tarnished by these lacks. For example, the Child Guidance Clinics of America from their earliest origins at the end of the first decade of this century suggested a real concern for children who were being improperly handled by society. It was often apparent, however, that over the years the rights of children in the whole treatment process were often subordinated to the needs of either parents, society, or the clinics themselves. As early as 1952, David Levy in his Academic Address to the American Psychiatric Association pointed out that child guidance clinics were often shaped to suit the needs of the professionals working therein rather than the specific needs of the children to be served. He stressed both the organization of child guidance clinics as well as their teaching functions and made it clear that the selection of patients for such services depended as much on the whims of the organization as on the clinical consideration of specific jobs that could be done for children. Very often the "intake" worker became an "extake" worker. Mental retardation, delinquency, and even unrecognized psychosis were categories that were systematically excluded from the clinic case load.

The very concept of collaborative therapy for children seemed to imply an individual concern for the child as a part of total care. At the same time he was separated from the restorative aspects of the family, a fact that became apparent much later as family therapy evolved. Parents who brought their children to such clinics wanted "something done for him." Usually this meant something to make the child conform to the parent's ideas of right or wrong, an idea which got translated into clinical concepts of health or unhealth. Throughout the history of the child guidance movement there was every evidence that, although clinical principles were followed, part of the job of the clinic was to fit the child into someone else's society rather than to look at society's need to be modified.

Following World War II there was a great increase in the number of residential treatment centers. Part of this was prompted by the recognition of more severe emotional disturbances in children and partly also by a growing need to separate out these disturbed children from the general population so that they would not be harmful to the larger society or even visible to that society. In many ways they therefore became the counterparts of detention centers and other methods by which society has removed children from their homes and put them out of view. At times, the operations of the largest of these treatment centers were no better than some of the penal institutions to which children had formerly been assigned by the courts. In fact, by collaborating with the courts, children who earlier would have gone to a detention center were placed in treatment without necessarily improving their lot. Institutional rules denied them contact with their families or, worse, the families abandoned them to long-term placement. One can, thus, make the case that adults were being protected from children by many of the services seemingly designed to be of assistance to the latter. Like the outpatient clinics, the residential services for children carried the promise of therapy and restoration. Often however, it appears that children were treated for long periods of time in order to make them fit into a mold designed by a conformist adult society. The processes of discharge suggested that the child could be freed from the institution only when he was willing to accept the constraints that society prescribed.

As patterns of clinical symptoms changed from the behavior problems of the earlier part of the century to the learning problems of the latter, the same interest in fitting children to society persisted. Schools became the major source of referral for children during the 60s and 70s. Learning problems appeared to be on the increase. A variety of theories for this was expressed. But in all instances the attempts at therapy were to make the child fit the systems of learning generally operative in the school systems. Although experimental ways of assisting children were used to achieve this end, the ultimate goal was to place the child back in a "normal" school where he would once more fit in with his peers and with the way the system functioned.

One of the most impressive by-products of development is the reaction of parents to any signs of independence on the part of the child. We are well acquainted with the manner in which both parents and society attempt to control and limit the activities of adolescence. We are less familiar with the same phenomenon when it occurs during the second year. At this earlier time the child is emerging from dependence and by his growth, his progress, and his strivings toward independence, threatens the comfortable situation of the parents. Many parents react at that time by becoming overly interested in the manners of children, in the discipline of children, and in the ways of teaching them behavioral patterns. All of these are designed in theory to help a child fit into society but many of them may be repressive in nature. At times discipline becomes highly coercive and even punitive. All this is done in the name of the child's "good." Thus controls are set up to protect the parental rights as well as to help children fit the system. Society in its efforts to do something about children very often sets up equal controls to protect adults from the aberrant or independent activities of children.

Equally, the legal rights of children have been ignored. In the legislative field, controls have been more obvious than supports. While the power of infants and children in homes may have seemed tremendous, the effect of this power on legislative and economic situations has been minimal.

In the deliberations of the Joint Commission on Mental Health of Children it became apparent that both strong commitments to services for children and a comprehensive approach to a health system were necessary. One of the impressive aspects of the studies of the Joint Commission reflected the powerlessness of children. The idea, therefore, of someone who would be an advocate for children seemed highly rational. Someone was needed to speak for, plan for, organize for, and pay for services and functions designed to enhance growth, to modify pathology, and to increase the wholesome and healthy functions of the psychologically disturbed or retarded child.

It is apparent that in planning any services that will benefit children we must avoid the pitfall of merely putting the child into a new kind of strait jacket appropriate to the community in which he lives. Rather the enhancement of the child's health should be primary. This leads to an important concern whether advocate services which would speak for the child's rights, his needs, and his health might not in themselves increase the dependent state of the child. The latter's efforts toward independence are often the causes around which services are organized. It becomes obvious therefore that certain advocates, both legal and clinical, must speak for this independence, must seek to enhance that which is health, and must not hide behind fear of such independence. Equally, however, the advocate must not become so powerful as to reinforce the dependence of those whom it is designed to assist. This is true of welfare advocacy, of legal advocacy, and of medical advocacy.

A variety of models of advocacy have begun to appear on the national scene. The legal model, expressed by the juvenile court is the oldest. Many individuals feel this has not fulfilled its ostensible function. Despite high hopes early in the century, many lawyers have opposed the concept of the juvenile court, feeling that the child does not obtain his classic rights at the Bar. The humanitarian aspects of the juvenile court are ignored by legal critics who feel that the system of law is often more important than the protection of the individual under the law.

The Gault case may very well be a landmark in the establishment of greater rights for children. In 1967, when this case reached the Supreme Court and a boy was freed from the State Industrial School in Arizona because of a highly improper trial, the Court declared that "neither the Fourteenth Amendment nor the Bill of Rights is for adults alone." It is very apparent that children have been essentially non-citizens, even though they appear to be protected pets. More often they are considered chattels. Many of the legal rights normally assumed by adult citizens are barred to them.

The early years of the 1970s have been notable for the appearance of a number of class action suits concerned both with the rights of patients in hospitals and of children in schools. In Alabama, the famous case of *Wyatt vs. Stickney* condemned the state hospitals for their standards, their care, and their concept of adequate treatment. Based on the due process clause of the Fourteenth Amendment, and utilizing also the "cruel and unusual punishment" clause of the Sixth

Amendment, the Court condemned the care of patients involuntarily committed to hospitals. It was a sweeping indictment of the state's institutions and resulted in some very profound political changes which at the time of this writing have not been resolved. A parallel case in Georgia, *Burnham vs. the State of Georgia,* suggested the very opposite; namely, that rights of treatment for patients were not the province of the Court. Both of these cases are currently in the appellate stage. Although broader than an immediate concern for children, the point of advocacy involved in these rulings applies to all children in hospitals who may or may not be getting adequate care and treatment.

Similar rulings from various courts, again not specifically directed toward children, have challenged the state's failure to pay compensation for institutional maintaining labor. This right of patients will also apply to children should the cases be adjudicated and made mandatory.

Perhaps the most notable class action suit involving children concerns the right-to-education for children in the state of Pennsylvania. There the verdict in *Pennsylvania Association for Retarded Children vs. the Commonwealth of Pennsylvania* stated that, since the laws of the Commonwealth demanded that children be in school, facilities must be provided for retarded children. Many states and communities attempt to provide such schooling. However, many children with various degrees of disability and handicapping are excluded from schools on the basis of arbitrary decisions making them ineligible for the services to which they are entitled. The ruling in *PARC vs. Commonwealth of Pennsylvania* is supported by a ruling, *Mills vs. the Board of Education of the District of Columbia.* Both of these suggest that since mandatory education is required in the various school districts a provision must be made for all children.

It seems likely that this form of advocacy will increase considerably. At the moment some of these rulings are extremely difficult to carry out and may serve as a deterrent to better care. Ultimately however, a rationality will be made out of these court decisions and an increase in rights for those previously denied may be demanded by the law as well as supported by the law. It will be important in understanding and carrying out these legal actions that once more a cloak of constraint does not deny the true legality and the true rights of the individuals involved. There will be strong political opposition to all of these legal procedures. Many of them will founder on the rock of finances as they have over the years. However, strong pressures on the part of parents and others who become professionally involved in advocacy for children may rescue and modify the procedures that are currently existing.

Recently, the phenomenon of the battered child has led to reorganized legal approaches to the health and social problems of children. Certain states, such as Hawaii, have developed complete health and legal approaches to the problem of the battered child, so that those individuals who are acting for the child, at times by taking him from the parents, are adequately protected. Such plans are advocacy-in-action related to a specific problem. By proposing and then utilizing various mandatory laws related to this syndrome they not only protect the medical and social agents who assist such a child, but also give evidence of a salutary approach to a specific type of advocacy.

Following the publication of the Joint Commission's report, "Crisis and Youth," Senator Ribicoff introduced S. 1414 to amend the 1971 Social Security Act by providing for the establishment of a child advocacy program. In May of 1971 a National Center for Child Advocacy was organized within the Office of Child Development. During that same year, Alfred Kahn of the University of Cincinnati began an intensive study of child advocacy programs. His project entitled "Child Advocacy Systems: a Baseline Study" identified the various activities labeled child advocacy throughout the country at various levels. In 1971 a Child Development Bill S. 2007 passed both Houses of Congress. It contained a specific proposal for local councils concerned with children's programs. This was vetoed by the President in December of 1971 but attempts are being made to write a new bill. The concept embodied in this bill was that of "operational advocacy." It called for a considerable restructuring and coalescing of resources. It mandated rearranging delivery systems so that present categorical activities of advocacy might be made more comprehensive. The Joint Commission had recommended that federal funding be provided for an advocacy system at every level of society. It strongly urged a National Advisory Council on Children, similar to the Council of Economic Advisers. It called for state child development agencies. It called for local child development authorities in cities and counties. It called for a network of child development councils throughout the nation. The inherent promise in these suggestions was that of an organized pattern of child care and advocacy for that care. The implication was that there needed to be representatives of services for children at all functioning levels of government in order that they not be forgotten, in order that their needs be looked at in the light of economic and political pressures, and in order that systems to carry out services for children be in some way functionally coordinated. This has proven the most difficult task.

At one level, advocacy is becoming evident in the field of early childhood education, especially infant education. Deriving from evidence of deprivation of children in the field of intellectual development, the Head Start program some years ago began to be developed as an advocate for children whose background put them at risk in the learning process. More recently, Parent-Child Centers designed to carry the teaching methods as well as the general health methods of Head Start down below the age of three, have provided an even more dramatic advocacy for small children.

The organization of these centers was initially planned to serve a relatively small number of children under the age of three in situations where health, education, and welfare services could be offered. Thirty-six Parent-Child Centers throughout the United States were established. Each was limited to 100 children with their parents. Various patterns of organization of these centers have been developed. All of them however carry the concept that the organization of services, especially those designed to enhance the health and knowledge of children, must include both parental teaching and child care. They represent a planned approach to child-rearing practices which has been notably absent from the American scene. We have a "non-system" of child-rearing and child development practices. These centers seek to develop a more adequate schema. Unfortunately this also raises the problem of government sponsored child-rearing methods, which is anathema to many in our population. Right-wing groups see the centers as violating their advocacy for home teaching. Actually the organization of the centers provides a service for children and parents who currently are getting no home teaching or adequate child-rearing care. The concept has been pushed further by the Office of Child Development into a home-based advocacy, "Home Start." This in many ways may be more appropriate to the American system of child-rearing.

The model of the Parent-Child Centers with involvement of parents in the educational and stimulatory aspects of child-rearing derives from medical and psychological knowledge and demonstrates the advocacy of a planned approach to child-rearing practices. The threat of such early child-rearing practices to right-wing groups suggests the potency of the advocacy.

In 1972, some of the federally funded Parent-Child Centers were designated as Child Advocacy Centers in addition to their major concerns about the education of small children. The objectives in adding the advocacy component included the further assessment of needs of children, better coordination of programs for children under five, identification of high-risk families, and the organization of a variety of services for children in these centers. The shift of these Parent-Child Centers to Parent-Child Advocacy Centers is still experimental. It was apparent, however, in the organization of the PPC's that they had become community centers for children or parents with very young children and that many services were beginning to attach to them in a realistic, if haphazard, fashion. The designation of the advocacy component reinforces what was already occurring and makes them more worthwhile.

For example, a Parent-Child Center established for children in the Boston area became located in what had previously been a settlement house. Other community agencies were working already in the same building. The center was offering educational and health services to children under the age of three as well as their parents. The parents brought in problems of older siblings which suggested the need for social and other welfare consultation. Some of these services were available through the other agencies. Others were added in the process of expanding the advocacy concept. Shortly it became apparent that a coalition of services was being organized around this one age group but serving the needs of older children in the same families as well as children yet unborn. More extensive health services were not available but health maintenance for the children enrolled in the program was an important consideration.

These programs can be viewed as an experiment. They currently demonstrate rather distinct educational stereotypes in their approach to the growing child. Knowledge garnered over the years from the field of dynamic psychiatry is less evident and the analytic developmental model is often ignored by the behavioristic advocates. A healthy blending of these various approaches to child-rearing still needs to be made in this area of infant education.

In the general field of health, there have been a variety of advocates for categorical care of children throughout the century. Organizations devoted to a specific aspect of health care are numerous. Groups concerned with mental retardation, cerebral palsy, tuberculosis, heart disease, etc., have been active advocates in organizing services and care for children. Some of these have been extremely effective. Their categorical nature, however, has diminished their effectiveness. They are vulnerable to legislative whim, both in giving and taking away funds. Truly advocated health care for children would demand a more organized pattern, preferably on a national scale, that would embrace not only the individual categories of childhood disability, but the multiple needs of all children in health, in mental health, and in intellectual development.

At the time of this writing a "mega-plan" has been suggested by the Department of Health, Education, and Welfare, in which funds will be given to the states on a revenue-sharing basis to cover all health or education or welfare needs of children. The logic of this flies in the face of the federally provided categorical grants. Those who have advocated a national categorical approach through grants will be annoyed by this counter-advocacy which suggests that the states can do better planning for the health needs as well as the educational needs of their children through a form of sharing from the federal government. The battle over this situation will pit advocate against advocate. This does not auger well for a healthy outcome for the ultimate consumer, be he child or parent.

Most recently, the National Institute of Mental Health and the Office of Education have offered grants to states and other national agencies to develop plans for broad advocacy within these jurisdictions. Interesting models have been developed in some of the state organizations. In Kentucky, for example, a model of case finding, publicity, and services that embraces the total needs of children within the state has been developed and will be experimentally funded. In Tennessee, a proposal has suggested that there be advocacy agents, not unlike the country farm agent, in many subdivisions of the state. Their primary concern would be the organization of all services for children within that corporate area.

Several of the national organizations concerned with the specific categorical needs of children also submitted proposals, but again these focused only on the unique needs of the child who suffers such a disability.

It is curious that we need advocacy for children. Their very helplessness and dependence along with the reward of their growth and their independence would seem to be adequate to force us to continually do appropriate things for them. The continuance, however, of childhood difficulties in all categories, including those in the field of mental health, suggest that either we are ignorant or that we are applying our knowledge poorly. One facet of advocacy suggests the need for coordination of knowledge and its application. It has bred in the past few years a variety of coalitions, consortia, and other systems pulling together organizations concerned with the needs and hopes of children. In such conglomerates may lie new hope for the child himself.

Most important in the field of psychiatry is the Consortium for Child Mental Health. Sponsored originally by the Academy of Child Psychiatry this has pulled together national organizations such as the Academy of Pediatrics, the PTA, and other organizations, to work in concert for better services for children. The push will include educating legislators and officials concerning the needs of children as well as expressing a strong concern about the organization of services. A parallel group is the Child Development Associate Consortium, representing primarily educators and child development specialists. This group seeks to develop standards for individuals who will carry out teaching procedures of young children. It hopes to utilize expertise, experience, and varying backgrounds of people in the total field of child development, as well as bringing together these diverse interests. Federally financed, it is preparing material to make possible the dream of a well-trained and certified "child development associate," able to cope with the multiple problems of assisting in this stage of the child's life. Members of the child psychiatry profession, represented for many years by the American Orthopsychiatric Association, welcome the idea of establishing a profession which will deal with individuals at a level where the care can be legitimately labeled preventive. Advocacy for prevention has been a cornerstone of American child psychiatry although it has not always been achieved.

Professional concern about children has often been the hallmark of individuals who are otherwise politically naive. More recently, it has become apparent that professionals, too, need advocates. This has led to enlisting the support of sympathetic legislators and jurists, not to make changes but to teach us how to make changes. Many of us have strong commitments, and yet the strength of our commitment sometimes isolates our advocacy. Isolated advocacy may at times have political clout but it does very little for the society as a whole. In fact it engenders competition where there should be comprehensive services. It engenders rivalry which does not necessarily build better products. It results in the separation of services for the existing clientele with the result that nobody gets anything.

An outstanding example of such competition was referred to earlier in the discussion of Parent-Child Centers. The emphasis in these centers became that of the educational approach, namely: teacher to pupil. The children in these centers were exposed to a variety of stimulating experiences as well as a variety of learning and cognitive experiences. Where such stimulation came in conflict with older theories of personality development the emphasis was on the educational approach. In one center the research and curriculum proposal suggested, "The PCC program on child care should avoid unnecessary controversies in areas that are tangential to intellectual growth, e.g., feeding, bathing, discipline." This statement would seem to epitomize the manner by which the curriculum developers have approached the idea of modifying lives of relatively small children. In the curricula derived from such cognitive theories of child-rearing the feeling was that the child should be treated firmly (if not harshly) during the early years so that an appreciation of the realities of life and the controls that are necessary to live in our society could be developed. The educational advocates who proposed these curricula and the intensive teaching that accompanied them, seemed uninterested in the advocacy that might have come from the students of personality development.

The missionary aspect of such advocacy omits a need for long range evaluation so dear to the medical, and hence, psychiatric profession. Despite the concepts of both Head Start and the Parent-Child Centers, there is no clear understanding as yet of how a child stimulated and enriched in the PCC and then carried on through Head Start will perform in public schools. In fact, the advocates of this early education suggest from their own observations that when these children do arrive at the doors of elementary schools, the educational systems are not prepared to cope with their potential advancement and thus the children regress. This is not because they have not gained something, but rather because the school system itself is not tooled up to their needs and capacities.

Another crucial aspect of many advocacy programs is that they neglect the basic culture of individuals for whom the programs are designed. Many new programs bearing the advocacy label are located in black ghetto areas of large cities. In such instances there may well be cultural values, previously present in the lives of the participants, that may or may not be considered in the planning of a new curriculum, new activities, and a new organization. One gets a very strong sense that classic middle-class values provide the general background for programs that are being thus offered. Indeed one finds that the participants very often actively lean toward these values and assume them very rapidly. Simple non-advocacy alternatives, enhancing the lives of individuals through direct payment, may very well be neglected by those who are pushing specific teaching, psychological, or health programs.

It was to organize the concept of advocacy at the federal level that the Office of Child Development planned, through an Interagency Panel, a unit called the National Center of Child Advocacy. Comprised of a Secretariat; a Division of Vulnerable Children; a White House Conference Follow-up Unit; and a Children's Concern Center, the prime Center coordinates activities described elsewhere in this paper. In addition, however, it lends support to many studies and operating plans within various parts of the federal system. Important to us as professionals and citizens, the Center is available to inform, to clarify, and at times to untangle efforts at local levels. Its resource functions may be, for many of us, its most valuable asset.

As an individual, a child does not like to be dissected and categorized. He needs a more concerted plan of approach. The needs for comprehensive services are great. The hopes of many will only be realized if the actions toward cooperative activity and advocacy are as potent as the size of the needs. Despite fervent hopes we have not attained a clear sense of being of help or service to the "whole child." A focus on advocacy, rather than on direct service, may make it possible to visualize the problem more clearly. Seen thus, we may surmount our avoidances, our denials, and our seeming rejection of the child in our midst.

3.

Purveyors of the Superego

THE REVEREND JOHN S. JENKINS

In America a popular concept of religion has been that its primary function is to make people "good." To a great degree, being "good" meant following the conventional morality while deriving inspiration and support by attending religious services. Usually the purpose of these services was to firm up our courage to fight for good against sin. Particularly among the members of the major Protestant denominations the result was that people were perceived as being divided into two groups—the good guys, who kept the moral code, and the bad ones, who did not. While the Ten Commandments were talked about a great deal as being the backbone of religion, the transgressions which created the greatest emotional stir usually were confined to the areas of alcohol and sex. To be sure, some people achieved a more sophisticated concept, but this often turned out to be not a different idea of religion but just a subtler idea of what sins were.

Instead of overt behavior, these people saw the real sins as envy, lust and pride. The function of religion remained that of using every means possible to keep the tendency toward sinful behavior and emotions under control.

Undoubtedly the primary restraint was the fear of social rejection of the offender. The cultic life of the religious group added its own incentives for obedience to the moral code. Protestantism and Roman Catholicism in the 19th and 20th centuries used the rewards of heaven and fear of hell as fully as possible. The baptismal service used by the Episcopal Church (although actually written early in the 16th century and being, in part, a translation from sources far older still) is illustrative, in many of its passages, of this emphasis. In the opening statement, the congregation is informed that none can enter the kingdom of heaven unless he is "regenerate and born anew." In one prayer, regeneration is defined as remission of sins. In the promises made by the one baptized or by the godparents, the person is asked to "renounce the devil and all his works, the vain pomp and glory of the world, with all covetous desires of the same, and the sinful desires of the flesh . . ." Finally, when the child is baptized, the priest makes the sign of the cross on the person's forehead "in token that hereafter he shall not be ashamed to confess the faith of Christ crucified, and manfully to fight under his banner against sin, the world and the devil."

Other rituals have conveyed much the same moralistic concept of religion, or at least have readily lent themselves, through portions of their phraseology, to the conveying of such concepts. In the prayers for the visitation of the sick, one calls for God to "sanctify the sickness . . . that the sense of the weakness may add strength to his faith and seriousness to his repentance . . ." The communion service opens with the awesome words "almighty God, unto whom all hearts are open, all desires known, and from whom no secrets are hid . . ." Immediately following that warning, the congregation rehearses the Ten Commandments. It does not take a scholar to see why the next thing in sequence is to cry: "Lord, have mercy!" The list of illustrations is endless. I have chosen these from the Episcopal Prayer Book, but the identical emphasis is to be found in both Catholic and Protestant traditions. The result of all this is that most adults today grew up thinking that the function of religion, like the police, is to keep us on the straight and narrow path. In psychiatric jargon, most 20th century people assume that the primary utilization of religion in life is as a purveyor of the superego. Popularizing theologians have for a number of years told us that the loss of this religious structure in our culture would result in a chaotic moral condition in society. I suspect this is a bit too simple.

Using rather loosely the Freudian concepts of id, ego and superego, I should like first to indicate that, historically, religions have served a much broader function than support for the superego in individuals and society, and then to turn to our contemporary scene for some speculations. I believe that even a superficial study of religions, ancient and modern, primitive and sophisticated, will reveal that usually the religious enterprise deals positively with all three areas of the Freudian trinity. To be sure, some periods in the life of a religious tradition seem to stress one aspect over the others, but the flowering of that tradition can usually be seen when there exists a somewhat equal expression of religion in all three aspects of the psyche. When the stress is heavily weighted in one direction, as the last two centuries have seen in the case of superego material, the results can be disastrous to organized religion and even to the culture that supports it. Let us now look at this matter more closely.

From our own rearing in this culture, it is obvious that religion has deeply influenced the superego structures of our society in terms of social ethics, and of the individual in terms of moral guidance. This aspect of religion is so obvious that many assume that this is all there ever was to the religious involvement in life. Images of the Protestant preacher denouncing sin and of Catholics lining up for confession are primary symbols of religious life in the recent past, familiar to all. That institutional religion should function in the superego of society at large may possibly appear less obvious, but the involvement of churchmen in the social strife of the sixties was tapping a tradition as old as the ancient prophets of Israel.

There have been religious traditions in which the involvement in superego function was practically non-existent. The fertility religions of Canaan, which Israel had to digest after conquering the land, are examples of this. Some of the popular mystery religions of the late Roman empire, such as the Attis mysteries, provide other illustrations. Both are significant because the first, Canaan, provided part of the environment in which the Hebrew religion took shape, and the other, the late Roman period, provided the environment in which Christianity emerged. As a result, the Hebrew-Christian traditions do, in fact, give heavy emphasis to the superego function of religion. However, superego was only one function of the religions of Judaism and Christianity. Both had borrowed a great deal from the religions around them. They used the material imaginatively, synthesizing it with their own strong ethical orientation. At first this took the form of law which was to regulate man's life in a righteous way, pleasing to God. The 15th Psalm is typical of this point of view. "Lord, who shall dwell in thy tabernacle? Who shall dwell in thy holy hill? He that backbiteth not with his tongue, nor taketh up a reproach against his neighbor."

Later, in New Testament times there emerged, as a result of the influence of Jesus, a bit more sophisticated superego influence. It was no longer to be a matter of the letter of the law, but true guidance for one's life was to come from a commitment to do good for another individual. A type of love developed, called *agape,* which, for our purposes, may be considered to be an affectionate, considerate regard for others in which the libidinal component is sublimated. The history of the development of *agape* in the piety and moral life of western Christendom is a fascinating story, but quite outside the scope of this paper. The final development or, rather, constriction of *agape,* Christian love, into a self-repudiating altruism is, however, not only a mutilation of the New Testament idea but also the final turn of the screw of an exalted and impossible superego demand that has contributed to the emotional stress of millions of people, and finally to the large scale abandonment of that kind of religion. The Hebrew-Christian tradition does, then, indeed have a deep involvement in the superego structures of our culture, but if religion were to be only a superego phénomenon,it would become lifeless.

Less familiar to the popular mind is religion's involvement in id phenomena. You will, I hope, forgive me for being somewhat vague, but religion, like poetry, is more caught than taught. I am not using the word id in a highly technical sense. For the purpose of this paper, let us consider it as a repository of raw energy, filled with potentialities. In our culture, it is very difficult to experience consciously and comfortably this aspect of religion. It has taken the writer twenty years of exposure to religion as a professional even to begin sufficient deculturization to find some expression of primal energy in a religious context. The truth, however, is that all great religions contain, and usually begin with, a primary involvement in the basic energy of life. Perhaps this is why religions always begin with myths and, further, why there is a good bit of common ground in the mythological structures of religions quite separate historically. Creation is always out of chaos. Chaos is often portrayed in the form of some amorphous beast, full of life but vague in description. Or, the undifferentiated mass is thought of as dark, watery and feminine, or perhaps androgynous. In the creation story of Genesis, we find that "the earth was without form and void; and darkness was upon the face of the deep." The word used for deep here is *tiamat,* the Babylonian primordial beast.

The act of creation is the interaction between this undifferentiated mass of energy and another entity, called in Genesis the Spirit of God, and in the Gospel of John, the *Logos,* or the Word of God. The latter is more enlightening. The Logos means communication. It means naming a thing (all of Chapter I of Genesis is naming). By naming, we call a thing into a precise existence, differentiating it from something else. We create order out of chaos. We mobilize and bind energy in form and give it specific expression. Creation is always a choice by the creator to bring into existence a *this* rather than a *that.* It is usually experienced as a gain (energy expressed), but also as a loss (to create or become a *this* rules out creating or becoming a *that.*) Another way to view *Logos* is as reason, or the rational. *Logos* becomes, like the ego, the selector, the planner.

In the poetic world of religion, primordial chaos, the source of life, has a strange quality about it. On the one hand, some contact with it must be maintained to keep the energy, the thrust of life, moving. Too much rationality and too much protection from the emphasis of raw energy, too much ego and superego, leave us with inadequate vitality. On the other hand the fascination with energy and life sometimes results in a pull toward the disintegration characteristic of the primordial. The mystics have always found a pull toward a loss of self almost as strong as the pull to participate in creation and being.

The cultural expression of religion is never static. It is a mistake to assume that the great preoccupation of the 19th and 20th centuries with superego function is a condition typical of Christianity in every century. One of the ways to tap something basic about life is through rhythm. Like alcohol (in small doses), rhythm has the capacity to unite the being of a person in such a way that we become an integrated expression of energy. Frontier religion has strong superego involvement, but equally as strong was an element given expression in the hand-clapping, foot-stomping and rhythmic singing. Cultic expressions like this are far more than innocent fun. They become, when combined with the ego, a religious experience in which something very basic about life is expressed. The ego, the *Logos,* gives it a name: knowing the Lord, getting the spirit, getting religion. It must be stressed that, while these experiences sometimes involved a spasm of the superego in the form of confession of sin, more often the sustaining nature of the religious life was such that the rituals became a unifying experience which gave energy, vitality and pleasure. The limitations of a specific self are momentarily suspended in a communion with the source of all life, called God. Thus frontier religion put one in touch not just with restrictive moral laws, but with an energy that gave courage and purpose to life.

Likewise, in previous centuries, the confessional did not dominate Catholic life. The ritual of the mass did. During those periods when men could really participate in the pageantry of the mass, they underwent a unifying experience which brought the ego and the id together in a powerful way, which the believer considered to be communion with God. The person experienced a wholeness as he adored the source of all life. Even more, he experienced a transcendence which brought him in contact with a power which left him courage and meaning. There was relatively little superego to it. I doubt if men will die for a God who is all superego. But one good, solemn high mass has often given more courage to face death than the rhetoric of a Patton.

The 20th century has witnessed a strange phenomenon, which I do not pretend to understand. What can be reported as fact is that, until recently, 20th century American religion had virtually abandoned the use of religious rituals as avenues to tap the vital energies of life. The essential use of the ego to give balance and reason to the expression of life's energy was also gradually removed from the theological world. Theology, rather than being the queen of the sciences, as Thomas Aquinas called it, faded from the university scene. The result has been the exclusive preoccupation of religion with superego functions. The Sunday School became a major symbol of religious life, and the Sunday School's primary function was to reinforce the basic moral teachings to which the family subscribed.

Some interesting consequences have ensued. Among them I would suggest the following: We have a tragic splitting of the psyche. The whole creation is one huge expression of energy, and man either stays in contact with that energy on some level or dies. No longer finding this contact in religious experiences, many have sought to grasp the battery in any way possible. Has there not been a growing sense of becoming frantic unless we "feel" something? We look for "authenticating experiences," "gut level" communications, and devices which 'turn people on.'" But when the superego is unintelligently related to the id, the ego suffers. In vain does the contemporary ego search for a meaningful philosophy with which to relate life's energy to reality structures. Under these circumstances, the mystic's intuition of a pull to nonbeing becomes quite understandable. In the desperate effort to stay alive, the threatened ego, abandoning an "irrelevant" superego, moves toward the primordial mass of undifferentiated energy. The result is not life, but disintegration. The promising avenues to energy such as violence and sex begin to dominate, but then ego has only raw energy, and can give it no name; there is no *Logos,* no integration, no part of a growing creation. Our senses become dull. Finally, even killing and fornicating are no longer fun, having long ago lost any relationship to meaning and integration of life.

The consequence of this development for institutional religion is obvious. Left with the dry bone of a superego no longer in contact with id or ego, it has no relevance. The results are everywhere to see, and need no further comment.

The decade of the sixties was the time when the shock of this development really came home to most of us. We are a frightened people. Sensing the disintegration of the ego and the meaningless expression of raw energy, many turn desperately to the superego to stop the process. Usually this is not an effort to integrate the ego meaningfully with the id, but just to stop the flow of raw energy. This is understandable and even necessary in times of panic when all is threatened. The movement toward superego may not succeed, but it is a major phenomenon of our times. Politicians are often elected on a law-and-order platform. Many other issues can safely be ignored. Felony squads quiet things down. Liberals are confused.

I believe that I have observed a similar trend among my psychiatric friends. Has this once rather liberal group moved, not only in politics but in the practice of healing, considerably toward a new emphasis on the superego? I wonder if some of the GAP reports of 10 years ago would be written similarly today? But you are better able to answer those questions than I.

In the field of religion a similar desperation swing to the superego has taken place. The most powerful religious movements of today are made of pure superego material. The Campus Crusade, the new fundamentalism, and the Jesus Freaks are examples. The mother of a daughter caught up in one of these movements told me, "I don't care what their theology is, just as long as they get her through her teens without her being on drugs or getting pregnant." In interviewing a number of the youngsters, I would have to agree that the rigid clamp-down on the expression of meaningless, destructive energy does indeed save some of them—at least for a while. Among traditional denominations also the lure of a heavy superego emphasis is felt. Those churches with plenty of people and lots of money are the same ones where sermons denounce long hair and promiscuity. The use of superego material of a past generation in these movements is totally unrelated to any effort to give the energy of life a meaningful expression. As a matter of fact, there is a tendency in part of this movement, especially the Jesus Freak, to drop out of society as much as possible. The anti-intellectual aspect of the movement is well illustrated by the new fundamentalism. Biblical fundamentalism is as dead in the theological world as hanging garlic around the neck of a sick person is in medical schools. Yet the new fundamentalism is one of the fastest growing religious movements of today.

A second type of religious reaction to the chaos of our time is an expression of energy and vitality in some ancient and rather extreme religious forms. The charismatic movement is illustrative. Anyone who attends a meeting where speaking in tongues is practiced cannot help but feel the vitality and pleasure that the participants express. One person expressed it as "getting my battery charged for all week." Another version of the same phenomenon is sometimes to be found in "knowing Christ." These people achieve a new sense of vitality. They believe that they talk to Christ and that He guides their life, even the minute details of it. He is their constant companion. For them, every day has little miracles in it. They have considerable euphoria in feeling that they are part of something big, and God is using them.

Both the charismatic movement and the Christ movement are primarily efforts to reach life's energy. At the same time, their members achieve a sense of peace and calm, because, unlike the drug approach, there is an inherited moral code in these religious forms. The energy has to be expressed in song, hand-clapping, or inwardly in mystic satisfactions.

In counseling a number of these people, I have found that, while there is vitality and energy expressed in the context of pleasure, it is usually unrelated to life within nature. It seems quite foreign to the world of lovers, of marriage, of child-rearing, of meaningful labor and the enjoyment of earth's pleasures. The expression of pleasurable energy in a moral framework brings a sense of security and peace. In the mind of the writer, it is bought at a very high cost—the withdrawal from the main currents of contemporary life.

All of these fear-driven returns to a strong superego may well help stop the disintegrative process at work among us, but they will surely bring no lasting peace. What is needed is a new integrative concept or ideal which will give valid expression of life's energy in the context of man's earthy life, organized by some reasonable understanding of man's purpose on earth, and channeled by restraints which naturally develop out of the wisdom of the experience. In other words, we need a new integration of the id, ego and superego. In the past, religion has been one of the major forces in life to assist in doing just that. Quite possible it will be again.

The new interest in the historical Jesus, emphasizing the humanity of man, is a promising movement. It has the double advantage of seeing the locus of life's energies squarely in the earthy instincts of man, and, at the same time, attempting to organize these instincts, needs and desires into a value pattern that is intelligently in touch with today's world. Jesus is seen not primarily as the Christ of faith, but as the man experienced by his contemporaries before they proclaimed Him Israel's Messiah. He is seen as man and as participating actively in the earthly concerns of men. He is keenly interested in social problems. He anguishes with the suffering. He rejoices at a wedding. He is tender with children. He is comfortable with women and crusty fisherman. He is capable of using force. He experiences doubt and uncertainty. His interest in life, his capacity to enjoy, is woven into a capacity for intimacy with others. He has found meaning in the quality of relationships. He developed a style of relationship which was something tender, sometimes painful, but always caring. He made people feel their worth because he had the capacity to bestow worth in the act of intimacy. His style becomes contagious. The excitement of the New Testament Church is proof of it.

The contemporary revival of interest in the humanity of Jesus affords us an alternative to the disjointed and separate utilization of superego material to calm the troubled seas. First, it finds in the earthiness of Jesus a new courage to face the basic instincts and needs of man rather than mutilate or abandon them. Growing up, being confused, having fun, experiencing the pleasures and the pains of nature, learning the dignity of meaningful labor, mating, birthing and child-rearing, gaining some earthy wisdom and learning the grace of diminishment—these are the content of life, the place where energy belongs. New prayers, contemporary religious music and liturgical changes all place these concerns squarely in the middle of the religious life.

Second, the movement finds an integrative power in the concept of love, of *agape,* as Jesus practiced it. It simply means that we are not whole, not truly human, until we recognize and participate in an interdependency with others. We must learn to open our lives, allow others to enter and to express caring. When this is done, we find purpose and fullness in extending ourselves into the lives of others. This interdependency in the concept of caring allows not only a freedom to express our very human emotions, but also a context in which the more destructive ones can be rendered less dangerous. In an atmosphere of caring, hostility, lust and pride can be recognized and then laughed at. The devil is never more helpless than when he is exposed and laughed at. The new movement shows promise in an ego development which integrates the basic energy of life into a meaningful whole. The revival of the ancient practice of passing the Peace is an illustration. Many are afraid of it, but when it works, it creates a joyful human exchange in the context of religion. People shake hands or embrace and greet each other in the name of the Lord.

Third, the superego of the movement emerges cautiously based on the revival of an ancient insight. St. Augustine once said that pure evil did not exist. What we saw as evil was a distortion or an abuse of the good. The basic characteristics of superego phenomena in the religious community I am describing is an effort to find the acceptable in man's transgressions before condemning the tragic and destructive side. The person who is always disruptive at meetings may be saying, "Please don't overlook me!" The adulterous person may be saying, "I am afraid of aging." If we reject the behavior swiftly and totally, we do not help ourselves or others in the fine art of maturing gracefully. Jesus searched for the good; he reinforced it, and the destructive behavior lost its appeal.

At a time when our society has a chaotic expression of energy, let us not hasten the disintegration by encouraging brutalizing and irrational superego patterns. Rather let the religionist and the psychiatrist have faith that we can once again find our way to an integrated psyche where the basic energies of life can be expressed in meaningful and beautiful patterns, guided by restraints intelligently formed and humanely administered.

4.

The Epidemiology of Mental Illness

JOHN J. SCHWAB, M.D.
and
RUBY B. SCHWAB

> Notwithstanding our advancement in general and medical knowledge, it must be confessed that psychology, or the science which treats of mental operations, is yet in its infancy. In reality, the reasoning faculties are but just emerging from the thraldom in which they have been alternately enchained, by the phantasma of superstition, the speculations of the ancient, or the scepticisms of modern philosophers. But because we know not what mind is, nor can explain the occult causes of its aberrations, we must not reject the evidence which observation furnishes, and opposes to supposition, on the event of insanity.
>
> GEORGE MAN BURROWS (1820) (1)

Psychiatric epidemiologists deal with the "evidence which observation furnishes" about health and disease in populations in the hope that this knowledge can be used for the treatment and prevention of illness in individuals and groups. In this paper, we will discuss some of the historic endeavors in this field as they relate to the problems which confront investigators today, look at some of the broad sociocultural processes—particularly a society's values—as they affect our thoughts and our work, and then offer a few suggestions about future directions for psychiatric epidemiology.

The groundwork for the epidemiology of mental illness was laid in the middle of the 17th century with the introduction of methods of quantification in the social sciences. As Paul Lazarsfeld (2) has pointed out, it is difficult for us to imagine the paucity of information available at that time and the difficulty of "obtaining numerical information on social topics." But enumeration and quantification were dominant ideas in the 17th century. For example, in the 1620s, Harvey's questions about the amount of blood that the heart pumped and his primitive calculation of the stroke volume led to the discovery of the circulation. In 1662 the first mortality tables were published by John Graunt, the originator of modern demography. Within a decade or two, Petty's "Political Arithmetic" was used to describe the characteristics of populations. And statistics, in the term applied to the enumeration of characteristics of the state (3), came into use.

Probably the first reference to the epidemiology of mental illness is found in Graunt's (4) "Observations on the Bills of Mortality." He wrote that: "The Lunaticks are also but few, *viz.*, 158 in 229250, though I fear many more then are set down in our Bills, . . ."

Simple records of admissions and discharges to mental institutions were compiled for administrative purposes. An example of these early records is supplied by John Strype's

(5) "Description of Bethlem Hospital." He found that between 1684 and 1703 there had been 1,294 admissions and that 890, or "two patients in three," had been cured and discharged—an enviable record.* A century later, Black's (6) analysis of the "Table of Cases" in Bedlam showed that of the 3,403 patients who had been treated from 1772 to 1787, 924 had been cured. In view of the relapse rate, Black concluded that the proportion cured was only one out of three—strikingly similar to some present-day statistics.

But during the last few centuries, interest in the epidemiology of mental disorders has fluctuated, stimulated during periods of social unrest by fears that mental illness was increasing. At the beginning of the 19th century, epidemiologic methods began to be used to determine whether mental illness was becoming more common. The social climate was seething with emotions aroused by the American and French Revolutions and industrialization. The great psychiatrists of the era chronicled the excitement. Benjamin Rush (7) wrote that: "The excess passion for liberty, inflamed by the successful issue of the war [American Revolution], produced . . . a species of insanity" which he termed "anarchia." And, Pinel (8) stated that the storms of the French Revolution stirred up "tempests in the passions of men, and overwhelmed not a few in total ruin of their distinguished birthright as rational beings."

To measure possible changes in the rates of mental illness, Richard Powell (9) studied the registers in England from

* The proportion discharged as cured excited Burrows (1), who in 1820, reported that the figures had been furnished by Dr. Tyson, the hospital's first physician. Burrows notes that, "this evidence is the more important, since it is half a century anterior to any quoted, either of this or any other institution . . . the recoveries were in a ratio, considering the then state of medical knowledge, surpassing perhaps that of most other diseases."

1775 to 1809. He concluded that insanity "was considerably upon the increase" in the ratio 100:129 between those years. There was widespread concern that the political turbulence and the complexity of civilization were too much for the capacity of man's nervous system. Sentiments of the time romanticized nature and the simple life and indicted civilization as the source of man's miseries. In his *Inquiry into Certain Errors Relative to Insanity,* in 1820, George Burrows (1) stated: "That this malady prevails more at one time than another is indisputable; but this is no proof of its increment." He believed that "mental derangement has been truly designated the vice of civilization," but after a detailed analysis of admissions into British asylums from 1775 through 1819, controlled for population growth, he reported that there had been only an apparent, not an actual increase in the number of insane. He attributed increased rates of admission in 1790-94 to deep sympathy about George III's mental illness, increased rates in 1800-04 to the failure of the harvest of 1800 and the "extremity of distress and suffering," and an increase in 1809 to the passage of a parliamentary bill for better care. Burrows concluded that the apaprent increase between 1775 and 1819 was produced mainly by two factors: first, the excited interest in the subject, and second, the improved facilities with more precise record keeping. These are factors which continue to influence our ideas about the prevalence of mental disorders.

In 1828 Andrew Halliday (10) conducted one of the first field studies after he found that the public records in Scotland showed only 648 patients in mental institutions and ten in jails. In words which presage our current thinking, he stated that those figures bore "no proportion to the actual number of insane persons in the kingdom." Then, applying a method which is still in use, he polled the 900 parishes in Scotland, obtained returns from 800 of them, and reported that the total number of insane was 3,700, of whom 1,861 were actually confined while the rest were wandering at large and begging.

In this country, about the same time, Amariah Brigham (11) declared that "we have no means of determining correctly the number of insane persons." In 1812, a committee in Connecticut had sent questionnaires to physicians and public officials in every town in the state to obtain accurate information about the number of mentally ill. They received 70 replies and concluded that there were 1,000 mentally deranged individuals, one for every 262 inhabitants in the state. Extrapolating from these figures, Brigham calculated that there must be 50,000 insane in the United States, a higher proportion than elsewhere in the Western world and a ratio which was at variance with the general notion that insanity was most common in England.

In the 1820's, Esquirol (12) said that "the question so often propounded for forty years presents itself: 'Is there now more insanity than existed previous to the [French] Revolution?' " He analyzed the records of admissions to the Bicêtre and the Salpétrière, compared the data with those gathered elsewhere in Europe and in the United States, and presented diagnostic classifications according to age, sex, and occupations. He noted that the number of insane in the mental hospitals in Paris had doubled within thirty years and emphasized that political commotions produced insanity "by changing the circumstances of all men"—either through misfortune or the sudden acquisition of wealth. But he concluded "that if the number of the insane has increased since the Revolution, that this augmentation is more apparent than real (13)." His conclusion was based on the comparative analyses of rates of admission to mental hospitals in various cities of France which showed "that this increase has no where taken place, except where the erection of buildings and improvements in their treatment have begun." He stated that this apparent increase was also due to the greater laxity in moral standards—a familiar note in our contemporary society which is attributing dissent, drugs, and disease to permissiveness.

Fears about a possible increase in mental illness, attributable to political turmoil and social change, thus prompted early epidemiologic studies. Results of the analyses of records of admissions to institutions and the data obtained from those early field studies were limited by the same problems which handicap psychiatric epidemiology today: (1) the inadequacy of such records; (2) the obvious limitations of rates-under-treatment data, recognized since Graunt's day and confirmed by Roth and Luton's (14) 1938 survey which showed that for every person treated for psychosis, nearly one psychotic had never been hospitalized; and (3) the problem of judgment in field studies which involves the definition of mental illness and the criteria for case finding.

With the growth and popularization of psychiatry since World War II, we are observing a renewed interest in the epidemiology of the mental disorders. In the midst of the third psychiatric revolution, as we are attempting to diagnose and treat the disturbed and the troubled in the community, the epidemiologist is challenged and perplexed, primarily by the difficulties in defining mental illness with exactitude. As Warren Dunham (15) explains, the definition of mental illness is being broadened. The widening of the definition may be responsible for the marked differences in the results of field studies conducted in the United States and northern Europe before and after World War II. Studies carried out in the 1920s and 1930s reported only about one-fourth to one-fifth as many cases as did those conducted after World War II. Although we cannot make direct comparisons between these studies because of differing methodologies, and, particularly, differing criteria for case finding, the percentages reported ill in studies before World War II ranged from 1.1 to 7.5% of the populations studied, in contrast to a range from 3.4 to as high as 60+% after the war.

Dunham maintains that a number of factors are responsible for the widening of the definition of mental illness. These are the development of office practice, frustration with the outcome of therapy with psychotics which led to a compensatory widening of the psychiatric net to include those who had "problems in living," and the greater availability of care. He concludes that the expanding definition has "served as a type of fuel" for the development of community psychiatry.

Repeated observations through the centuries do indicate that an expansion of facilities is associated with their increased use and with the recording of greater numbers as mentally ill. However, we think that the widening of the definition of mental illness, the expansion of treatment facilities, and the community based mental health movements are *all* reflections of more fundamental social processes. On the contemporary scene, the accelerated rate of social change, the growth of population, and the proliferation of technology are accompanied by alterations of roles and the disappearance of traditional norms. As a result, individuals and groups have difficulty evaluating their anxieties and behaviors and are likely to categorize as illness any or all of those which are painful or troublesome. Also, illness is a more socially desirable label than deviance; the "ill" person is not wholly responsible for his actions, and there is always hope that medical science will find a cure for illness.

Furthermore, a society may *need* to relegate a certain percentage of its population to special roles, for example, the sick role, if not to institutions. In order to assess thoughts at this level of abstraction, we must place them in a historical perspective.

Evidence of society's seeming need to exclude a certain segment, the undesirable, for whatever reason, is supplied by Foucault (16) in his book *Madness and Civilization.* He points out that, as leprosy vanished in Western Europe at the end of the Middle Ages, mental illness increased. England and Scotland, with a population of 1,500,000, opened 220 leprosaria in the 12th century; in the 14th and 15th centuries practically all of them were closed because of lack of patients. In France, 1,200 lazar houses existed at one time, but late in the 17th century, only a few lepers could be found to be lodged in the houses reserved for that purpose. Foucault maintains that although leprosy disappeared, the values and images persisted. The values and images attached to the leper and the social importance of his exclusion were transferred to witches, to the mentally ill, and later, to the poor. As the medieval period drew to a close, vast epidemics of mental illness erupted. Hecker (17) attributes the "mental plagues" of the 15th and 16th centuries to the great natural disasters, adverse social conditions, and also, to a disposition of mind peculiar to the Middle Ages. As Foucault (18) indicates, "madness was given a place in the hierarchy of vices [and was linked not] . . . to the world and its subterranean forms, but rather to man, to his weaknesses, dreams, and illusions."

During the next few centuries various means were used to extrude, eliminate, or immure the disturbed and the undesirable. In the 15th century the ship of fools had transported the deranged away from the medieval cities. And in that century and the next, hundreds of thousands of witches were exterminated. But in the 17th century, with the decline of witchcraft, which had served as a dominant means of social control for more than 200 years, walled institutions were substituted for bonfires. A few years after the founding of the Hôpital Général in Paris in1656, it held 6,000 persons, around one percent of the population (19). By the end of the 18th century, there were 126 workhouses (bridewells) in England. An entire network of centers of confinement spread across Europe; these hospitals, houses of correction, and prisons contained the insane, the felons, the beggars, and other deviants who were thus excluded from society. The confinement of the 17th century, according to Foucault (20), marked a decisive event in the history of unreason: "the moment when madness was perceived on the social horizon of poverty, of incapacity for work, of inability to integrate with the group."

The historical record has profound implications for the epidemiology of mental disorders; the varying definitions and standards of mental health and illness reflect Western society's values, particularly its tolerance of deviance and nonconformity. Schneider (21) mentions that: "The major 'cause' of mental disease is seen as some form of disorientation between the personality and society." From looking at history, we can see that the "some form of disorientation" involves norms and especially values, as well as disturbances of the mental faculties. Consequently, as the psychiatric epidemiologist approaches his work today, he encounters the problem of how to conceptualize and define what he is attempting to measure. This is a necessary task which must be accomplished before mental illness can be measured; but it is a seemingly insurmountable difficulty since the definition of mental illness has been dependent on society's changing standards and values, not on objective, consensually agreed upon criteria.

As a basis for defining mental illness, the medical model has had limited utility, although it can be used for diagnosing and classifying a few of the more clear-cut psychiatric syndromes. In his essay on "Health as a Social Concept," in which he advocates the medical model, Aubrey Lewis (22) points out that social disapproval cannot be considered as a criterion of mental disorders because disapproval is a function of the values of both the group and those who make the judgments. Likewise, he dismisses nonconformity as a criterion of illness since it is usually expressed in terms of social role and is influenced by conflict, culture lag, and social change. Lewis emphasizes the importance of the evaluation of the patient's total performance and insists that, "the criteria of health are not primarily social: it is misconceived to equate ill health with social deviation or maladjustment (23)." He outlines the medical model as consisting of three traditional types of data: (1) the subjective—the patient's complaints, (2) the objective—some disorder of function which is apparent to an observer, and (3) the typological—the conformity of the symptoms and signs to a recognizable clinical pattern.

In contrast, social scientists emphasize impairment, rather than illness. As Nagi (24) indicates, it is taken for granted that disease involving "active pathology" obviously produces impairment, but that not every impairment is the result of disease. An implicit assumption is that some impairments are traceable to sociocultural causes. Impairment is viewed as deviance from the norm, deficiency in role performance, or distance from the "ideal" character type in a given society.

Durkheim (25) recognized the tautology inherent in the traditional definition of health as adaptation and illness as maladaptation. In outlining objective rules for distinguishing between the normal and the pathological, he equated health with the average for a given society at a given time in the course of its evolution. He said:

> We shall call "normal" these social conditions that are most generally distributed (a statistical norm) and the others "morbid" or "pathological." If we designate as "average type" that hypothetical being that is constructed by assembling in the same individual the most frequent forms, one may say that the normal type merges with the average type, and that every deviation from this standard of health is a morbid phenomenon . . . each species has a health of its own, because it has an average type of its own. . . . The healthy constitutes the norm par excellence and can consequently be in no way abnormal.

Definitions of mental illness derived from either of these models are inadequate for purposes of case finding. The medical model implies that mental illness is a discrete state of the organism. Logically, this leads to concepts of health and illness as entities—as vastly different conditions—and to a disregard of the human being in whom health and illness coexist. Furthermore, the symptoms and signs of the mental disorders are so widely and variably distributed that the sufferer and the observer have difficulty evaluating them in the absence of clear-cut standards and criteria. Even the professionals cannot agree about the syndromes; Cooper (26) has recently shown that almost all the large differences in hospital admission diagnoses are "artifacts due to differences in the diagnostic practices of the psychiatrists and differences in the recording systems." Also, the attempts to apply the medical model have led to an abuse in modern medicine—"either-or" dichotomization and the diagnosis of mental illness by exclusion. In this respect, we should recall that in the *Malleus Maleficarum,* Sprenger and Kraemer (27) outlined tenuous guidelines for the differential diagnosis between natural disease and witchcraft. If the presence of "extrinsic causes accompanied by bad humors in the blood or the stomach" could not be established, then witchcraft was considered to be the cause of the trouble.

The social science model, implying the presence of a hypothetical standard of health, the average for the society, emphasizes the relativity of health and illness. A definition of mental health derived from this normative model is difficult to use for case finding during periods of rapid social change and shifting standards. Logically, it leaves little or no room for an appreciation of individuality and the uniqueness inherent in human variation. Also, criteria of mental health based on proximity and conformity to social norms are paradoxical in the case of the sick society. Scott (28) expresses this point succinctly: in some more absolute sense, conformity to the norms of a sick society would, in itself, "constitute mental illness." And, when carried to its logical conclusion, the normative model may be dangerous—it could be used to brand all deviance, dissent, and nonconformity as illness.

In addition to the limitations of these two basic models, just the disparity between them handicaps the epidemiologist, who, as a creature of his time, is seeking objective criteria for measuring mental disorders while he is aware that they always arise in a social setting and thus reflect the group's values as well as its standards. Felix and Bowers (29) insist that, in actuality, case finding is a function of the community rather than the clinician. Engel (30) has noted that "considering the tremendous variability of life circumstances, it should perhaps occasion surprise that any consistent clinical syndromes can be identified."

The difficulties in defining mental illness and in identifying cases are described poignantly by Machado de Assis (31) in his story, "The Psychiatrist," written in the 1890s.

> In the 18th century, a highly esteemed psychiatrist in a Brazilian province was empowered to build a mental hospital. In order to find scientific criteria for selectively admitting those who were mentally ill, he studied laboriously, reviewing the works of the great physicians, philosophers, and theologians. He concluded that mental disorder was evidenced by a disturbance of reason or of the mental faculties, a deviation from Aristotle's "golden mean." With scientific objectivity, he thereupon institutionalized all who manifested such imbalance. This was a painful task, personally, because he had to include many whom he had known and liked. But even after a large group was confined, social unrest and deviant behavior were still noticeable. He broadened his criteria and admitted greater numbers until a majority of the population was hospitalized. Then he reevaluated his criteria and decided that perhaps the mentally ill were the remaining few, those who appeared to be balanced despite the chaos of the times. Accordingly, he released the first group and incarcerated

> the latter, the minority who had displayed moderation in all things. However, this was not a solution; social unrest, behavioral aberrations, and psychic distress were still prevalent. Realizing that scientific precision had not been achieved, with supreme logic, one night he released all of the inmates and institutionalized himself.

In view of the controversy about and the limitations of traditional models of mental illness, in our epidemiologic study of a southeastern county, we are measuring social psychiatric impairment (32-34). We were led to the conceptualization of social psychiatric impairment by an increasing recognition that all illness arises in a social setting, that it is culturally defined, that differential rates of illness are associated with sociodemographic factors, such as income, and that broad sociocultural processes are linked to both availability of treatment and type of therapy received. The concept of social psychiatric impairment extends beyond the limitations of a medical model of illness by including the subjective, interpersonal, and larger social ramifications of personal distress, of behavioral disorders with their interpersonal consequences, and of deviance with its societal implications.

Our concept of "social psychiatric impairment" encompasses psychosocial distress along four dimensions: (1) traditional definitions of psychopathology, reported as the presence or absence of symptoms; (2) levels of functioning at home, at work, and in the broader social arena; (3) the quantity and quality of interpersonal relationships; and (4) indices of aspiration and satisfaction.

A second major problem confronting the psychiatric epidemiologist relates to the difficulties of studying the characteristics of the environment in the modern world where the environment is not only man-made, but also, is primarily a social one. Furthermore, in view of the evidence (35) that our biological and social systems are, in reality, closed ones (that there are limits to growth), we should heed Hinkle's (36) statement about the necessity of taking a "unitary view of the man-environment relationship." Because of the interrelatedness of the host and the environment, it is seemingly impossible to isolate independent variables. Theoretical scientists freely acknowledge that the investigator always influences the experiment. Furthermore, in conceptualizing the universe according to general systems theory (a metaphor of our technological era), we cannot plausibly explain how an investigator can be simultaneously inside and outside of the interacting systems, whether they are open or closed ones.

Psychiatric epidemiologists have focused their efforts on searching for associations between rates of disorder and the sociodemographic characteristics of the afflicted. In our epidemiologic study of a southeastern county, the major hypotheses center on the possible relationships between rates of social psychiatric impairment and the extent to which certain groups participate in and derive benefits from the rapid rate of social change which is occurring.* Those who are unable to obtain the benefits, because of physical, cultural, or other handicaps, or those who are out of phase with the rate of change, can be viewed as experiencing deprivation or personality conflict and therefore are marginal, vulnerable groups in whom we would expect to find high rates of impairment.

* As McKinney and Bourque (37) have shown in their article "The Changing South: the National Incorporation of the Region," the rate of social change in the South has been more rapid than elsewhere in the nation, particularly during the last two decades.

Of the pretest random sample of 322 respondents interviewed in their homes, 31% were rated as impaired. The impairment rates were higher in the blacks (39%) than in the whites (28%); in the women (35%) than in the men (23%); and in the widowed, divorced and single (ranging from 38-46%) than in the married (26%). The relationship between age and impairment was curvilinear, higher in those under the age of 30 (37%) and over the age of 60 (37%) than in those in the 30-59 age groups (27%). We found the usual relationship between income and impairment; 49% of those with annual family income of less than $3,000, and 42% of those with incomes from $3,000-$5,999 were impaired; but impairment rates declined to about 15% in higher income groups. As expected from the associations with income, the impairment rates were significantly higher among service workers or laborers than among those engaged in professional, technical, and managerial jobs. With one exception (the curvilinear relationship between rate of impairment and age), these findings are consistent with reports from most community studies of mental disorder.

Preliminary analyses of the data from our random sample of 1,645 adult respondents confirm the pretest finding that the most statistically significant relationships are between low socioeconomic status and high scores on our depression scale (38) and also high scores (in the "caseness" range) on the Leightons' Twenty Question Health Opinion Survey (39).

Associations between higher rates of illness and poverty were observed by Burrows (1) in both England and France in 1820. In his analysis of the "alleged causes of disease," Pliny Earle (40) stated in 1848 that pecuniary difficulties and want of employment were the most common. And associations between higher rates of mental illness and lower social class status are the single most consistent finding in numerous community studies during the last 40 years (41). To explain this association, investigators are trying to determine to what extent either social causation or social selection is responsible for the greater prevalence of mental disorders among the poor and the underprivileged (42,43).

But in limiting efforts at explaining the prevalence of mental disorders among the poor to testing hypotheses about social causation and social selection, we may be overlooking the historic issue—values. The Protestant Ethic, dominant in Western society for almost 400 years, exalted work. At various times during the last few centuries, poverty, once regarded as a Christian virtue, has been equated with criminality and sin. In his *History of the Bloomingdale Asylum,* in 1848, Pliny Earle (44) mentions repeatedly that numerous patients were admitted from and removed to the Almshouse, apparently shunted back and forth between the mental institution and the poorhouse. The persisting influence of the Protestant Ethic on definitions of mental illness, as well as institutionalization, is evidenced by Reid's (45) 1960 statement that we may have to accept an operational definition of mental disorder "as a disturbance of feeling or behavior which is disabling enough to cause admission to the hospital or an *inability to work effectively.*" [Italics ours.]

In view of the growing tendency to categorize many types of deviant behavior as illness, some of the habits and customs of subcultural groups which are at variance with standards of the dominant society are being regarded as impairments produced by mental disorders. Such judgments are made from a frame of reference which does not include, for example, characteristics of the culture of poverty. For instance, missing work may be judged as evidence of serious impairment according to our work-oriented middle-class standards, when, in reality, it may be a subcultural norm. Foucault (46) notes that during the 17th century: "The new meanings assigned to poverty, the importance given to the obligation to work, and all the ethical values that are linked to labor, ultimately determined the experience of madness and inflected its course."

Another major problem which challenges the psychiatric epidemiologist is that the manifestations, forms, frequency, and distribution of illness not only vary from culture to culture but change through time in a particular culture. Changes in the incidence, prevalence, and types of disorders appear to accompany rapid social change produced by innovation and the proliferation of technology. The rapid rate of social change and culture lag entails gains and losses for groups and individuals, alters role obligations and expectations, and requires adjustments and adaptations which appear to influence the frequency and distribution of diseases.

In our study, from an analysis of impairment rates controlled for age, sex, race, and income, we can project in terms of probability the characteristics of those least likely and most likely to be impaired (47). Typically, those showing low rates of impairment are men in the age group 30-60. They have been educationally prepared for change and reap its benefits by working at professional, technical and managerial jobs and receiving commensurate incomes. They are newcomers to the community. Their life styles are consonant with the rate of social change—characterized by mobility, a high degree of interaction with friends, and little contact with relatives. They are at home in Suburbia, U.S.A.

Thus, they are participating in and appear to be in phase with the rapid social and cultural change.

The vulnerable groups, showing high rates of social psychiatric impairment, are: the young adults and the elderly; the unmarried, especially the widows and the divorced women; either those who have resided in the county more than ten years or those who are hypermobile; and generally, the poor, many of whom are black. Although some are isolates, with the exception of the young most are in close touch with their families and desire to see them frequently. We conjecture that these kinship networks are used for support, enabling the vulnerable and the impaired to cope or to compensate for their unpreparedness for social change. Their low incomes are evidence of marginality if not deprivation in a rapidly changing society which emphasizes affluence and the consumption of material goods. These groups are not sharing in the benefits of change and they appear to be out of phase with the rate of change.

In *Psychosocial Medicine,* James Halliday (48) documents the marked shifts in the sex ratios, as well as the changing frequencies of various psychosomatic illnesses in the first half of this century. For example, peptic ulcer, mainly a disease of women in the 19th century, became primarily a male affliction in the middle of the 20th century, although the male-female ratio is now changing from 4:1 to about 2½:1 (49). And, syncope, once common (and an appropriate social response), now occurs rarely. Of 1,628 respondents in our community study, only seven women and one man reported that they had fainted during the preceding year. Hill (50) has recently noted that certain common characteristics of schizophrenia and gross manifestations of involutional melancholia have been disappearing during the last twenty years. As patterns of illness change, therefore, the epidemiologist must continually revise standards for judging and measuring the mental disorders.

Moreover, epidemics of mental illness, once considered to be relics of a bygone era, are reappearing on the contemporary scene. In 1943, Schuler and Parenton (51), in reporting an epidemic of hysteria among high school girls, noted that descriptions of such phenomena were common during the 19th century, but that they had not been able to find a single publication on mental epidemics in the United States for the past forty years. During the last few years, however, an increasing number of epidemics of hysteria, myalgia nervosa, and even mass anxiety about fears of insect bites have been reported (52-54). The latter is frighteningly reminiscent of the epidemics of tarantism which prevailed in the late Middle Ages.

There is some evidence that mental disorders spread by contagion. Hecker's (17) research on the outbreak of the Dancing Mania, which eventually afflicted thousands and affected entire communities until the beginning of the 17th century, found that it began with the revels of St. John's Day in July, 1374. His work showed that those strange disorders, as well as mass outbreaks of hyteria, spread by "morbid sympathy" until they became real epidemics. In the midst of societal change, he said that these diseases were spread "on the beams of light—on the wings of thought." Recently, in addition to evidence from the analyses of epidemics of mental disorders in the 1950s and 1960s, Winklestein's (55) studies provide further proof for contagion. He found that the blood pressures of nonrelated persons living in the households of hypertensives were higher than matched controls.

Redl (56) has indicated that mental contagion does not develop unless there are social restraints to be reduced. This insight helps to explain that mental disorders become epidemic not only when social conditions are conducive, but also, when repression is excessive. From this point of view, the epidemics of hysteria in the Victorian era can be seen as miscarried revolts against the sexual repression of that time. This gives us concern about whether the increasing sociopolitical repression in the United States will lead to mass outbreaks of mental and behavioral disorders, outbreaks which now can be transmitted quickly and easily by our mass communication systems.

This discussion has outlined some of the conceptual and methodologic problems hindering the work of psychiatric epidemiologists. The strictly methodologic include the serious inadequacy, as well as the variability of records, and they overlap with the more fundamental ones which hinge on the conceptualization and definition of mental illness. With the exception of a few clear-cut syndromes, such as those produced by genetic defects, the organic brain syndromes, process schizophrenia, and manic-depressive psychosis, mental illness is socioculturally defined and thus the label "mental illness" expresses a society's values. As a reflection of a society's values, the definition not only changes from era to era, but apparently contracts and expands. This variability handicaps the epidemiologists' case finding efforts which are burdened further by the changing frequencies and forms of mental illness and its appearance as epidemics. These thoughts are not offered to suggest that mental illness is a myth, but rather to emphasize the profound influence of sociocultural forces on all of our ideas and behaviors, including those which we designate as health or illness.

Fears about increased mental illness accompanying political commotions and social unrest at the end of the 18th century sparked the first epidemiologic studies. Interest in the epidemiology of mental illness now parallels our awareness that we are living in an era of accelerated social change. Epidemiology, in Morris' words, "the Cinderella of the medical sciences" (57), made immense contributions to knowledge about illness and health care long before microbes were identified as the necessary causes of the infectious diseases. Those contributions were the result of painstakingly slow, accurate observations and the application of methodologic strategies. They were not achieved by prematurely attempting to reach definite conclusions nor by drawing causal inferences from inadequate or non-representative data. As Malamud (58) has emphasized, "the determined search for a single cause and a quick remedy" has doomed much psychiatric research.

To increase its scientific contributions, psychiatric epidemiology now needs to base its efforts on three approaches. First, we need descriptive epidemiology which focuses on phenomenology and is content at this time to accumulate basic information about symptoms and syndromes, their frequency, distribution, manifestations, and variations. In the standard textbooks of psychiatry, authorities on the mental disorders state repeatedly that there are no reliable data and, indeed, little or no knowledge available about the frequency and distribution of the various neuroses and personality disorders and only limited information about the psychoses (59,60).

Second, the information obtained from descriptive epidemiology should be interpreted only from a perspective which includes the frank recognition that our ideologies and values are dominant influences. They will determine our judgments and our biases about mental illness unless we make them explicit and acknowledge their historic relativity in our pluralistic society.

Third, we need to maintain a humanistic orientation to give meaning to the epidemiology of mental health and illness, which, in essence, is the study of the expression of emotions in all their variability. Karl Jaspers (61) has said that: "If we get a concrete knowledge (of the mental illnesses which are undesired variations of human life which require treatment) some light is thrown in its turn on the psychic disorders of organic origin. Human life is involved at every point, the concepts of the natural sciences are indispensable but here do not suffice and everywhere we find a gulf between man and beast."

REFERENCES

1. Burrows, G. M.: Is Insanity an Increasing Malady? *An Inquiry into Certain Errors Relative to Insanity; and Their Consequences; Physical, Moral, and Civil.* London: Thomas and George Underwood, 1820.
2. Lazarsfeld, P. F.: Notes on the History of Quantification in Sociology: Trends, Sources, and Problems. *ISIS,* Vol. 52, Part 2, 1961.
3. *Ibid.*
4. Graunt, J.: Natural and Political Observations Mentioned in a Following Index, and Made upon the Bills of Mortality (1662), in Hunter, R. and Macalpine, I. (Eds.): *Three Hundred Years of Psychiatry.* New York: Oxford University Press, 1963, pp. 166-167.
5. Strype, J.: Description of Bethlem Hospital, in Hunter, R. and Macalpine, I. (Eds.): *Three Hundred Years of Psychiatry.* New York: Oxford University Press, 1963, pp. 306-310.
6. Black, W.: A Dissertation on Insanity: Illustrated with Tables and Extracted from Between Two and Three Thousand Cases in Bedlam (1810), in Hunter, R. and Macalpine, I. (Eds.): *Three Hundred Years of Psychiatry.* New York: Oxford University Press, 1963, pp. 644-647.
7. Rush, B.: Quoted by Hunter, R. and Macalpine, I. (Eds.): *Three Hundred Years of Psychiatry.* New York: Oxford University Press, 1963, p. 821.

8. Pinel, P.: *A Treatise on Insanity*. New York: Hafner Publishing Co., 1962.
9. Powell, R.: Observations upon the Comparative Prevalence of Insanity at Different Periods, in *Medical Transactions*. London: Longman, 1803, p. 139.
10. Halliday, A.: A General View of the Present State of Lunatics, and Lunatic Asylums, in Great Britain and Ireland, and in some Other Kingdoms (1828), in Hunter, R. and Macalpine, I. (Eds.): *Three Hundred Years of Psychiatry*. New York: Oxford University Press, 1963, pp. 785-788.
11. Brigham, A.: Remarks on the Influence of Mental Cultivation upon Health (1832), in Hunter, R. and Macalpine, I. (Eds.): *Three Hundred Years of Psychiatry*. New York: Oxford University Press, 1963, pp. 821-825.
12. Esquirol, J. E.: A Treatise of Insanity (trans. 1845), in Goshen, C. E. (Ed.): *Documentary History of Psychiatry*. New York: Philosophical Library, Inc., 1967, p. 354.
13. *Ibid.*, p. 355.
14. Roth, W. S. and Luton, S. H.: The Mental Health Program in Tennessee. *Amer. J. of Psychiat.*, 99:662, 1943.
15. Dunham, H. W.: Community Psychiatry, in Kiev, A. (Ed.): *Social Psychiatry*, Vol. I. New York: Science House, Inc., 1969, pp. 217-237.
16. Foucault, M.: *Madness and Civilization*. New York: New American Library (Mentor Books), 1967.
17. Hecker, J. F. C.: Epidemics of the Middle Ages, 1833 (trans. by B. G. Babington). London: Woodfall and Son, 1844.
18. Foucault, M.: *Madness and Civilization*. New York: New American Library (Mentor Books), 1967, p. 30.
19. *Ibid.*, p. 47.
20. *Ibid.*, p. 61.
21. Schneider, E. V.: Sociological Concepts and Psychiatric Research, in *Interrelationships Between the Social Environment and Psychiatric Disorders*. New York: Milbank Memorial Fund, 1953.
22. Lewis, A.: Health as a Social Concept. *The State of Psychiatry*. New York: Science House, Inc., 1967, pp. 179-194.
23. *Ibid.*, p. 194.
24. Nagi, S. Z.: Some Conceptual Issues in Disability and Rehabilitation, in Sussman, M. B. (Ed.): *Sociology and Rehabilitation*. United States: American Sociological Association in cooperation with the Vocational Rehabilitation Administration, U.S. Department of Health, Education and Welfare under VRA Grant No. RD-1684-G., no date, p. 100.
25. Durkheim, E.: *The Rules of Sociological Method*. London: Collier-MacMillan, Ltd., 1938.
26. Cooper, J. E.: The Use of a Procedure for Standardizing Psychiatric

Diagnosis, in Hare, E. H. and Wing, J. K. (Eds.): *Psychiatric Epidemiology*. New York: Oxford University Press, 1970, p. 119.
27. Quoted by Zilboorg, G., in *A History of Medical Psychology*. New York: W. W. Norton & Co., 1941, p. 159.
28. Scott, W. A.: Research Definitions of Mental Health and Mental Illness, in Bergen, G. and Thomas, C. S. (Eds.): *Issues and Problems in Social Psychiatry*. Springfield, Ill.: Charles C. Thomas, 1966, pp. 109-133.
29. Felix, R. H. and Bowers, R. V.: Mental Hygiene and Socio-Environmental Factors. *Milbank Memorial Fund Quarterly*, 26:125, 1948.
30. Engel, G. L.: *Psychological Development in Health and Disease*. Philadelphia: Saunders, 1962.
31. Machado de Assis: *The Psychiatrist and Other Stories*. Berkeley and Los Angeles: University of California Press, 1966, pp. 1-45.
32. Schwab, J. J., McGinnis, N. H. and Warheit, G. J.: Toward a Social Psychiatric Definition of Impairment. *British J. of Social Psychiat.*, 4:1, 51-60, 1970.
33. Schwab, J. J. and Warheit, G. J.: Evaluating Southern Mental Health Needs and Services: A Preliminary Report. *Florida Medical* J., 17-20, January, 1972.
34. Schwab, J. J., McGinnis, N. H. and Warheit, G. J.: Social Psychiatric Impairment: Racial Comparisons. *Amer. J. of Psychiat.*, 130:2, February, 1973.
35. Abelson, P. H.: Editorial in *Science* commenting on D. H. Meadows, *et al.*: *The Limits to Growth*, 175 (4027):1197, 1972.
36. Hinkle, L. E.: Relating Biochemical, Physiological, and Psychological Disorders to the Social Environment. *Arch. Environ. Health*, 16:77, 1968.
37. McKinney, J. C. and Bourque, L. B.: The Changing South: National Incorporation of a Region, *Amer. Sociol. Review*, 36:399-427, 1971.
38. Warheit, G. J., Holzer III, C. E. and Schwab, J. J.: An Analysis of Social Class and Racial Differences in Depressive Symptomatology: A Community Study. Presented at the Annual Meeting of the American Sociological Association, New Orleans, August, 1972. Accepted for publication to *Journal of Health and Social Behavior*.
39. Schwab, J. J., Warheit, G. J. and Holzer III, C. E.: Mental Health: Rural-Urban Comparisons. In *Proceedings of the Fourth International Congress of Social Psychiatry*, accepted for publication.
40. Earle, P.: *History of the Bloomingdale Asylum*. New York: Egbert, Hovey and King, 1848, pp. 20-21.
41. Dohrenwend, B. P. and Dohrenwend, B. S.: *Social Status and Psychological Disorder: A Causal Inquiry*. New York: Wiley and Sons, 1969.
42. *Ibid.*
43. Dunham, H. W.: Social Causation and Social Selection Theories of Schizophrenia: A Methodological Analysis, in Masserman, J. H. and Schwab, J. J. (Eds.): *Social Psychiatry*, Vol. I. New York: Grune and Stratton, to be published in 1973.

44. Earle, P.: *History of the Bloomingdale Asylum.* New York: Egbert, Hovey and King, 1848, pp. 20-21.
45. Reid, D. D.: *Epidemiological Methods in the Study of Mental Disorders.* Geneva: World Health Organization Public Health Papers, No. 2, 1960, p. 31.
46. Foucault, M.: *Madness and Civilization.* New York: The New American Library, Inc. (Mentor Books), 1967, p. 61.
47. Schwab, J. J., McGinnis, N. H. and Warheit, G. J.: Social Change, Culture Change, and Mental Illness. In De la Fuente, R. and Weisman, M. N. (Eds.): *Proceedings of the V World Congress of Psychiatry.* Amsterdam, The Netherlands: Excerpta Medica, in press.
48. Halliday, J. L.: *Psychosocial Medicine: A Study of the Sick Society.* New York: W. W. Norton, 1948.
49. Schwab, J. J., McGinnis, N. H., Norris, L., and Schwab, R. B.: Psychosomatic Medicine and the Contemporary Social Scene. *Amer. J. of Psychiat.,* 126:11, May, 1970.
50. Hill, J. D. N.: Quoted by LeRiche, W. H. and Milner, J. in *Epidemiology as Medical Ecology.* Baltimore: Williams and Wilkins Co., 1971, p. 315.
51. Schuler, E. A. and Parenton, V. J.: A Recent Epidemic of Hysteria in a Louisiana High School. *J. of Social Psychol.,* 17:221, 1943.
52. Friedman, I. T.: Methodological Considerations and Research Needs in the Study of Epidemic Hysteria. *Amer. J. Public Health,* 57 (11): 2009-2011, July, 1967.
53. McEvedy, C. P. and Beard, A. W.: Royal Free Epidemic of 1955: A Reconsideration, *Brit. Med. J.,* 1:7, Jan., 1970.
54. Champion, F. P. and Taylor, R.: Mass Hysteria Associated with Insect Bites. *J. So. Carolina Med. Assn.,* 59 (10):351, Oct., 1963.
55. Winkelstein, W.: Cited by D. M. Spain, Discussion: Sociocultural Factors in Chronic Organic Disease. *Ann. N. Y. Acad. Sci.,* 84:1031, 1960.
56. Redl, R.: The Phenomenon of Contagion and "Shock Effect" in Group Therapy, in Eissler, K. R. (Ed.): *Searchlights on Delinquency.* New York: International Univ. Press, 1949.
57. Morris, J. N.: *Uses of Epidemiology.* London: Livingston, 1957.
58. Malamud, W.: Research in Schizophrenia, in Usdin, G. (Ed.): *Psychiatric Forum.* New York: Brunner/Mazel, 1972, pp. 16-26.
59. Arieti, S. (Ed.): *American Handbook of Psychiatry,* Vol. I. New York: Basic Books, Inc., 1959.
60. Friedman, A. M. and Kaplan, H. I. (Eds.): *Comprehensive Psychiatry.* Baltimore: Williams and Wilkins, 1967.
61. Jaspers, K.: *General Psychopathology.* Chicago: University of Chicago Press, 1963, p. 790.

5.

Changing Trends in Psychotherapy

JUDD MARMOR, M.D.

Most psychiatric historians trace the beginnings of dynamic psychotherapy to the currents initiated by Mesmer in the late eighteenth century, currents which made the first substantial inroads into the then prevailing approaches based on somatic supremacy. By the time Freud opened his office in Vienna in 1886, a considerable development was already beginning to take place in the treatment of neurotic disorders. The Nancy school under Bernheim had coined the term "psychotherapeutics," and strongly emphasized the importance of suggestion in the treatment process. Under the influence of this school, a variety of psychotherapies were developed over the next decade by French psychiatrists, all emphasizing techniques of suggestion, persuasion, and indoctrination. Pierre Janet described unconscious psychodynamic mechanisms and developed a system which he called "psychological analysis." In Switzerland, Paul Dubois achieved considerable prominence and success with a method that he called rational psychotherapy, in which he specifically abjured "authority, suggestion, and suggestibility" which he considered to be only of temporary effect. He believed in "curing the will through self-education," and his method was based on modifying "the erroneous ideas that the patient has allowed to creep into his mind." He recognized, he said, "but one means of education, persuasion by means of proof, by demonstration, by logical induction, and by reason which touches the heart (1)."

Thus the method of treating neurosis that Sigmund Freud gradually evolved in the 1890's and early 1900's was not entirely a unique one. His special genius was that in addition to a well-organized therapeutic method, he also evolved an original and creative psychological theory resting on developmental concepts. He was the first to emphasize the importance of sexuality, especially infantile sexuality, in human behavior, and the first to recognize and identify the significant phenomena of transference and countertransference in the psychotherapeutic process. Freud believed that most psychoneurotic disorders could be traced back to the experiential vicissitudes of the first six years of childhood, and his psychoanalytic method was based on the assumption that if patients could be enabled to recall and "work through" the repressed memories of these early experiences, they would *ipso facto* be cured of their disorder.

It is an ironic paradox that Freud, who more than any other man in history, is credited with shattering man's belief in his rationality by emphasizing the degree to which man is driven by blind, irrational forces outside of his awareness, nevertheless put his own ultimate faith in man's reason. "We may insist as much as we like," he wrote, "that the human intellect is weak in comparison with human instincts, and be right in doing so. But, nevertheless, there is something peculiar about this weakness. The voice of the intellect is a soft one, but it does not rest until it has gained a hearing (2)." Freud regarded the analytic treatment of neurotics as a process whereby "the consequence of repression [is replaced] by the results of rational mental effort (3)." "Where id was, there shall ego be (4)."

It is worth noting that despite the sometimes bitter disputes that have arisen between the Freudian and other psychoanalytic schools of thought—from the earliest Adlerian and Jungian variations through the diverse neo-Freudian groups, to the current Kleinian vogue—this basic premise of Freudian psychotherapy has never really been seriously questioned by these other schools. Differences have been principally over what constituted the best or most "correct" interpretation of the underlying psychodynamics, but all psychoanalytic schools have shared the assumption that making the correct cognitive interpretation to the patient is the core factor in the therapeutic process.

As the years have passed, however, the classical psychoanalytic model has undergone a number of modifications, and the sharp line of demarcation between psychoanalysis and other forms of dynamic psychotherapy has become blurred (5). Although there are still some who adhere rigidly to the original therapeutic technique recommended by Freud, more and more psychoanalysts have begun to modify their techniques in a number of ways. Thus they often see their patients two or three times weekly, instead of four or five. Many more patients are seen sitting up, with less rigid insistence on the use of the couch. Relatives are interviewed and occasionally even seen conjointly with the patient instead of being strictly excluded as they were formerly. In contrast to the old dictum that no major life changes were to be permitted for the duration of the analytic process, many analysts not only allow their patients but even encourage them to make basic changes in their life patterns when these changes seem rational and constructive. Finally, many psychoanalysts have begun to feel freer in general to enter into active communicative exchanges with patients instead of remaining bound to the classical incognito "neutral mirror" model of relative silence and impassivity.

One important consequence of this trend toward increasing flexibility in technique has been a growing interest in the *process* of the psychotherapeutic transaction, in contrast to the former preoccupation with its ideational or verbal content. Research into the nature of the psychotherapeutic process (6,7,8) has begun to make it increasingly clear that although cognitive understanding as administered via interpretive psychodynamic "insight" is a valuable adjuvant and facilitator of therapeutic change, it is by no means a *sine qua non* for such change. Considerable evidence has accumulated to indicate that the psychotherapeutic process is a learning process; what is most relevant to this process, however, is not so much specific historical correlations between past experiences and current reactions, as it is the acquisition of new models of behavior, thinking and feeling. Moreover, these new models are not always achieved cognitively and consciously, but as often as not are acquired subtly, as a result of overt or covert suggestion, unconscious identification with the therapist, corrective emotional experiences in the interaction with him and a kind of operant conditioning via implicit or explicit expressions of his approval or disapproval. In this process, the nature and quality of the patient-therapist interaction, the real personalities of both patient and doctor, and the degree of faith, hope, trust, and motivation to change that the patient brings to the therapeutic situation are of paramount importance in enabling the new learning to take place successfully. These factors obviously also encompass the transference and countertransference aspects of the psychotherapeutic relationship. It should be noted, too, that in contrast to the early views of psychotherapy in which the patient was regarded as an essentially passive object to whom the therapist applied certain objective skills and powers, the newer views take cognizance of the active and mutual transaction between patient and therapist.

Contemporaneously with the growing awareness on the part of many dynamic psychiatrists of these learning aspects of the psychotherapeutic process, a major new trend in psychotherapy, explicitly rooted in theories of learning, began to make its appearance in the 1950's. The best known of these was Wolpe's "reciprocal inhibition" therapy, based on the assumption that if anxiety-provoking situations or phantasies were associated with complete muscular relaxation, the anxiety would be inhibited and the capacity of the situation to provoke anxiety would be rapidly extinguished (9). Wolpe's reported successes by this technique quickly brought in its wake a host of other technical psychotherapeutic innovations, all presumptively based on Pavlovian, Hullian, or Skinnerian theories of conditioning behavior. Aversive conditioning techniques of many types, operant conditioning methods utilizing varying forms of reward and punishment, desensitization, social reinforcement, training and rehearsal techniques, and the like have been developed and reported in great profusion, all claiming a high rate of success.

It is worth noting that most of these techniques, in contrast to the dynamic psychotherapies, tend to eschew cognitive awareness. The emphasis in them is strictly on altering behavioral manifestations, and the subjective problems, feelings or thoughts of the patient are considered, if not unimportant, at least irrelevant to the psychotherapeutic process.

Still another major trend in psychotherapy also began to emerge in the 1950's—a trend which focused *neither* upon cognitive awareness, *nor* upon behavior, but rather on the *feeling states* of the patient. Perhaps the earliest exemplar of this approach was Carl Rogers, who advocated a technique of therapy based primarily on reflecting the patient's feelings back to him (10). From these modest beginnings a wide spectrum of techniques has gradually emerged, designed to heighten emotional awareness and encourage the expressions of feelings. These techniques are usually employed with groups, and involve such approaches as sensitivity training, so-called gestalt therapy, as well as various forms of bodily contact, and marathons—nude or otherwise—all designed to break down both rational and conventional controls, and to intensify emotional and sensate experience. The past decade has seen an enormous profusion of public offerings of such therapies, some leaning heavily on erotic overtones, others moving toward transcendental meditation, Zen, Yoga, and the like.

A more recent trend which represents a kind of marriage between the scientism of the behavioral techniques and the inward focus of the feeling-oriented therapies has been the proliferation of therapeutic approaches based on bio-feedback mechanisms and aiming at the relief of anxiety by the promotion of the relaxation thus achieved.

However, all this does not even begin to exhaust the list of therapeutic offerings that have emerged in the last few decades. I have referred above to the diverse group settings in which many of the feeling-oriented therapies have taken place. But group therapies in themselves have occupied an important role in the psychotherapeutic armamentarium for the past 25 years at least, and have been used within psychodynamic frameworks, as well as behavioral ones. Analytic group therapy has been conducted within Freudian, neo-Freudian, and Kleinian orientations; other approaches have invoked psychodrama, sociodrama, transactional game-therapy, and behaviorally-oriented role-playing or rehearsal in groups. There have been small group and large group therapies; conjoint marital therapies, and multiple marital groups; single family and multiple family groups; groups for adolescents, for the elderly, for divorcees, for parents without partners, for accident-prone individuals, for drug addicts, for alcoholics, for criminals, for people with sexual inadequacies, and for homosexuals.

The 1950's also witnessed the dramatic emergence of Dianetics, initially as a hoax, then as a fantastic merchandising operation when to its founder's surprise the public took it seriously. After a few years of widespread popularity it underwent a rapid demise, only to reemerge a decade or so later in the pseudo-religious garb of Scientology, under which it is experiencing a mild renascence. A somewhat related approach presently enjoying some popularity on the West Coast is Primal Scream Therapy, which also employs the technique of regression (not to the intra-uterine state, as in Dianetics,—merely to the moment of birth!) but combines it with an emphasis on the noisy release and dramatic acting out, in both dyadic and group settings, of presumably buried early infantile angers and anguishes.

These latter approaches, of course, are variations on the abreaction theme in psychotherapy, based on Freud's early belief that the release of repressed childhood memories with their attached affects would bring about a discharge of fixated libido that would automatically cure the patient. Freud abandoned this approach when he found that the abreaction effect was only a transitory one, and replaced it with the more tedious, far less dramatic, technique of "working through" resistances. The dramatic appeal of a sudden cure by abreaction, however, continues to hold sway in the popular mind, and reappears periodically not only on stage and screen, but also in a variety of therapeutic techniques like the foregoing. The sudden and rapid "cures" (where are they all now?) of lifelong personality disorders by LSD and other psychoactive drugs (the amphetamines, the barbiturates, CO_2, etc.) in 5 or 10 dramatic sessions, that were being widely reported a few years ago, were based on the abreaction hypothesis also.

Quite a different approach which has achieved some popularity in recent years is the so-called reality therapy of William Glasser. This technique ignores unconscious and developmental psychodynamic factors and places great emphasis on conscious personal responsibility for one's actions. It is a kind of "Dutch Uncle" approach to psychotherapy and is a throwback to the exhortatory and persuading techniques of the 19th Century. Originally employed in relationship to adolescent delinquents in a controlled environment where it proved useful, it appears quite simplistic when Glasser attempts to apply it to the understanding and treatment of severe psychoneurotic and psychotic disorders.

* * *

It should be quite apparent, even from this cursory survey, that the past 25 years has witnessed the emergence of an enormous array of psychotherapeutic techniques, each with its own group of devoted adherents, and each trumpeting its superiority over all others. What are we to make of them?

It seems to me that despite the enormous profusion of psychotherapeutic techniques that we have been witnessing in the past few decades, a careful look at what has been happening will reveal that the pattern is not as haphazard as might appear on first sight. Indeed, there is reason to surmise that the character of these therapies is related to certain significant trends in our contemporary culture, trends that are operating simultaneously, even though often at cross-purposes.

The first of these is a strong current of anti-intellectualism—a current which has been described in detail in Roszak's *The Making of the Counter-Culture* (11). This is, I believe, a reaction to a widespread disenchantment with, and unconscious fear of, the results of scientific technology. The increasing complexity and tensions of urban life, the pressures toward conformity imposed by standardized mass comunication media, the background menace of nuclear annihilation and ecological spoliation,—these and other factors beyond the scope of this paper all have contributed to a mounting sense of helplessness, alienation, and distrust of science and technology in large numbers of the American people. It is not surprising, therefore, that psychotherapeutic techniques have arisen which are responsive to these feelings, and that these techniques have flourished expansively. Particularly representative in this regard are the various sensitivity-type group therapies, all avoiding cognitive insights, and focusing instead on emotional expressiveness and physical contact (with or without erotic elements). Also part of this trend have been the therapies based on transcendental meditation and on Eastern philosophies (a rejection of the "technological West"). Thus it is not accidental that we usually find both the sensitivity groups and the Eastern philosophy approaches offered at the same "Institutes." Another expression of this anti-intellectual pattern is the extraordinary resurgence of astrology, with its combination of quick psychological diagnosis and facile psychotherapeutic guidance. Numerology, witchcraft, and spiritualism are other aspects of the same trend which have been reappearing. Perhaps it is unfair to put parapsychological research in the same category inasmuch as a number of sincere and dedicated scientists have been devoting themselves to a legitimate exploration of this field. Nevertheless, the emotional pull of this field for many of its devotees stems from a similar search for answers beyond the realm of science and bordering on the supernatural.

The second major contemporary cultural current stands in direct contrast to the one just described. It is the remarkable advance in technological and communicative techniques as they apply to the sources of human behavior. As might be expected, many therapists have seized on these technologies and have attempted to adapt them to the modification of human behavior. Thus we have witnessed a growing use of tape recorders, movies, videotapes, computers, and various electro-therapeutic devices. Growing sophistication concerning psychopharmacological agents has led to their increased use also as adjuvants to psychotherapy. Presently bio-feedback techniques are being widely developed to facilitate control of both voluntary and autonomic nervous system mechanisms.

The third, and in some ways the most farreaching in its ultimate effects, of the major cultural factors impinging on psychotherapeutic change has been the rapidly burgeoning societal demand for more economical and more equitable distribution of health care, along with the shortage of trained professional personnel to meet this demand. As a result there has been increasing pressure on the psychiatric profession to abandon its emphasis on costly long-term one-to-one psychotherapeutic techniques, and to replace them with more economical short-term or group approaches.

Psychoanalysis found its earliest applications in the treatment of middle and upper class individuals, primarily because only they could afford such therapy. It found a receptive haven, and enjoyed its greatest popular acceptance, on American soil, despite Freud's derogation and distrust of this country, because only an affluent nation such as ours could afford to cultivate and utilize so expensive a technique on a broad scale. It is ironic to note that in a way it was precisely the success and popularity of psychoanalytic psychiatry in the United States both during and after World War II that paved the way for the forces that began to undermine it in the succeeding decades. As the mental health movement grew stronger, and more and more people became aware of what dynamic psychotherapy could offer, there was an increasing demand for such treatment from people of more modest means. This became an important factor in the tendency of analytically trained psychiatrists to begin seeing patients fewer times weekly, and to begin experimentation with short-term therapies as well as with group therapies. (After all, it may not be unfair to speculate that Freud's insistence upon daily visits with his patients may have been at least partially influenced by the fact that in the initial years of his practice he had a great deal of open time in his schedule!)

The point is, of course, that both theory and practice, in any field, are never independent of their socio-cultural milieu, and what we are witnessing today in psychotherapy is that profound socio-economic pressures are rapidly modifying its forms and modes of operation.

The advent of third-party payments, for example, has had a major impact by bringing insurance companies and governmental agencies into the picture as standard-setters and evaluators for psychotherapeutic practice. Despite the fact that the two major national psychoanalytic organizations—the American Psychoanalytic Association and the American Academy of Psychoanalysis—are making valiant efforts to have psychoanalytic therapy included in any national health insurance program, the sheer logic of cost analysis makes it highly unlikely that a technique involving 4-5 expensive visits per week for an indeterminate (and sometimes "interminable!") number of years can be included in such a program. At best any viable insurance program will have to set some fiscally tolerable limit on the number of psychotherapeutic visits per year that it can subsidize, and that limit will almost surely be considerably below a 4-5 time per week, 50 week per year frequency.

It may be argued that this will represent a serious loss for psychiatry and will deprive some patients of the opportunity to achieve maximum or optimum therapeutic benefit for their problems. The bias of my own psychoanalytic training might lead me to lean somewhat in this direction. And yet in all candor I am forced to admit that such a conviction is more an article of faith than a matter of fact. I know of no satisfactory hard data to suport the conclusion that long-term 4-5 time a week psychoanalytic treatment produces superior ultimate results in terms of emotional growth and motivation than does long-term 2-3 time a week analytically oriented psychotherapy. Indeed, at least as far as the treatment of certain phobic and sexual dysfunctional disorders is concerned, the present evidence seems to be that some behaviorally-oriented procedures of relatively short duration are considerably more effective than standard psychoanalytic treatment.

On many grounds, therefore, it seems safe to predict that the coming decades will see a continuation of the trend to more active, shorter-term psychotherapeutic techniques, as well as an expanding use of group therapies. As experience has grown with group therapy, both on a short-term and long-term basis, it has proven to be a highly effective technique for mobilizing behavioral change, and, of course, it has the advantage of lowering unit-costs as well as of making more efficient use of psychotherapeutic person-power. This is not the occasion for a discussion of the indications and contraindications for group therapy versus individual psychotherapy. Each approach has therapeutic values which are indicated in specific instances, and at times both may be indicated. What we shall be seeing more of, therefore, as time goes on, I suspect, is the expansion of a trend that has already begun, that is, of combining individual with group therapy. More and more young psychiatrists are acquiring skills in both modalities and are able to use either technique or both as the indications call for them.

Indeed, many psychiatric residency programs today are training their graduates to be capable of utilizing a broad-spectrum psychotherapeutic approach encompassing behavioral *as well as* psychodynamic techniques, in both individual and group contexts—although there is still much to be desired in this respect, particularly with regard to conjoint marital and family therapies.*

Obviously, in some instances alternative therapeutic options may be available, since some patients can be equally helped by diverse approaches. In such cases the therapist's choices of technique will continue as now to be determined in part by his own idiosyncratic characteristics—his training, his professional identification models, as well as his personality make-up and system of values—which make him feel more comfortable with some approaches than with others. Also it is only fair to point out that it is highly unlikely that any one psychiatrist can be expected to acquire superior skills in all psychotherapeutic techniques.

I believe that behavioral therapy methods are here to stay, but that as time goes on, its practitioners will become increasingly aware of the interpersonal and subjective variables operating between them and their patients, and will be able to incorporate these variables in their approaches. Some behavioral therapists, such as Lazarus and his students, have already moved in this direction (12).

By the same token, dynamic psychotherapists will no longer, in justice to their patients, be able to continue to ignore the short cuts to symptom-amelioration offered by behavioral techniques, and will have to learn to make use of them when indicated. Thus we can anticipate, in the

* See Martin and Lief, *Resistances to Innovation in Psychiatric Training as Exemplified by Marital Therapy* in this volume, p. 132.

decades ahead, techniques that will attempt to combine the two basic approaches into new technical forms. Behavior therapists like Brady (13), Marks and Gelder (14) have begun to attempt this, as have dynamic therapists like Feather and Rhoads (15). The latter two therapists have recently reported on a method of ingeniously combining psychoanalytic concepts with behavior therapy by desensitizing, not the external anxiety-producing stimuli—as is usually done in behavioral therapies—but rather the underlying unconscious conflictual drives and impulses from which the patient's symptoms are presumably derived. Their reported successes certainly merit further explorations along such lines.

I would predict also that the taboo on the adjunctive use of psychopharmacological agents that has characterized the practice of many psychoanalytically oriented psychiatrists will become a thing of the past. This is not to say that some of the concerns upon which this taboo was based were without merit. The too liberal use of such agents can all too easily become an avenue toward narcotizing patients into a deceptive kind of anxiety-free apathy without the therapists' having to face up to the more difficult task of helping their patients learn to cope more effectively with their life problems. It can also serve to mask emotions which need to be worked through therapeutically, or to facilitate denial or avoidance reactions on the part of the patient. On the other hand, there is no doubt that excessive anxiety or depression on the part of a patient may consitute an impenetrable obstacle to psychotherapy, and it is both inhumane and inefficient to allow such patients to continue to suffer because of a blanket therapeutic taboo against the use of medication; the judicious use of medication in properly selected cases, far from interfering with the psychotherapeutic process, can facilitate it.

It would be too much to expect that the present profusion of polymorphic therapies will not continue in the future, although we can anticipate that those fringe therapies whose results are essentially dependent on the placebo effect of their novelty will be dropped by the wayside as this effect wears off. However, they will almost inevitably be replaced by new ones, promising equally miraculous results. The hope for magic is a deeply rooted one, and so long as there are unscrupulous purveyors who are willing to promise such magic, there will be an ample supply of purchasers! Conceivably, however, the regulating power of governmental and insurance agencies in the decades ahead may serve as a brake on some of the more extreme therapeutic approaches by refusing to honor them for payment.

One of the most significant shifts in psychiatric theory and practice that has been taking place in recent decades has been the increasing recognition of the importance of the milieu in both the production and the amelioration of psychopathology. This has resulted in a shift from the previous, psychoanalytically influenced, primary preoccupation with intrapsychic factors to an examination and inclusion in the therapeutic program of other factors in the life system of the individual. Thus we have witnessed not only a movement toward the inclusion of "significant others" in the psychotherapeutic process in the form of conjoint marital therapy and family therapy, but also the entire trend toward community psychiatry with its emphasis on modification of environmental factors wherever possible. In recent years it has become fashionable in some circles to deprecate the community psychiatry movement as promising more than it can deliver, and as tending to minimize intrapsychic considerations in mental disorders. Both points are legitimate criticisms. Intrapsychic mechanisms cannot and must not be ignored in any approach to psychopathology, and there have indeed been foolish excesses in some community psychiatry programs. But the basic premise of the community mental health center concept—to make mental health delivery systems visible and geographically and economically accessible to all people—is a sound one and should not lightly be discarded; neither should its corollary premise, which rests on systems theory and recognizes the important interrelationships between man's inner and outer worlds, and the need to make changes in both, if preventive psychiatry is ever to become a reality.

This brings me finally to still another major aspect of the current and future psychotherapeutic picture. Even prior to World War II, the development of mental hygiene centers resulted in the beginning use of allied mental health professionals, particularly social workers and psychologists, in the mental health delivery system. After the war, the indication for psychiatric care gradually expanded from its previous emphasis on the care of psychotics and severely disabled neurotics, to a concern with the mental health needs of the entire population. Under the emerging concept of the "right to treatment," programs have been established for the treatment of school problems, alcoholism, drug abuse, mental retardation, geriatric problems, and criminal behavior; and non-psychiatric physicans, psychologists, social workers and nurses, to say nothing of occupational and recreational therapists, special educators, probation officers, vocational, pastoral and marital counselors, have become part of the mental health "team" and are making positive contributions to it. More recently, as part of the community mental health program, new groups of so-called "paraprofessionals" and "indigenous mental health workers" have also been enlisted and trained to function within the mental health delivery system.

To further complicate the problem, increasing numbers of these non-medical professionals have elected in recent years to leave the clinical and institutional settings, and have moved out into practice to do various forms of psychotherapy.

It is greatly to the credit of the members of the psychiatric profession that, after an initial period of resistance to this incursion upon their "territorial rights," they are gradually coming around to a recognition of the fact that the realities of this nation's mental health needs are such that the involvement of non-medical professionals is both essential and inevitable. Increasing numbers of psychiatrists have begun to participate in the training of these allied groups, as well as to work on various programs involving cooperation and collaboration with them. Within the past year the Assembly of District Branches of the American Psychiatric Association has endorsed payment under medical insurance plans to non-medical health professionals provided "their services are rendered as part of a plan of treatment that is supervised and/or prescribed by a physician."

One can only guess at what the long-term consequences of these developments for the future practice of psychotherapy by psychiatrists will be. There is, of course, a possibility that economic factors, such as lowered third-party payments, may function to gradually exclude psychiatrists as the primary providers of psychotherapy, utilizing them only as diagnosticians, consultants, and supervisors of such care. This would mean that people who wanted psychiatrists as their primary psychotherapists would have to pay for such care outside of any governmental or private insurance programs. I consider such a development to be unlikely, however.

I cannot conceive of state or federal governments, or of the rest of the medical profession for that matter, condoning the deliberate exclusion of a medical specialty from a major segment of its medical function. Moreover, I do not believe the public would accept such a denial of their right to receive psychotherapeutic help from whomever they considered best qualified to give it to them. One could argue that those who wished to see psychiatrists could supplement their insurance payments to meet the higher fees of the more highly trained professional. Another possibility, however, is that insurance payments for psychotherapy may be graded on the basis of the professional qualifications of the psychotherapist. It is a fact that the psychiatrist is the only one among mental health professionals presently qualified *not only* to do psychotherapy, but also to make a differential diagnosis, to prescribe medication or somatic therapy, and, if need be, to hospitalize a patient for treatment.

There has been an interesting development in just the last few years that may be pertinent to all this. After almost a decade in which applicants for psychoanalytic training had been steadily decreasing, there has been a gradual resurgence in their number. I do not believe this is because an increasing number of young psychiatrists have decided to devote themselves to formal psychoanalytic practice. All of the evidence is that these young men and women are as interested as the rest of their contemporaries in all of the new technical developments in psychotherapy as well as in community psychiatry. I believe, rather, that this trend is due not only to the fact that they are recognizing the importance of understanding one's self as the basic instrument in all our psychotherapeutic techniques, but also that, when all is said and done, they are realizing that the mere proliferation of techniques in psychotherapy is not enough. In the final analysis, psychotherapy without any rational underpinning and understanding of underlying psychodynamics tends to become a kind of shot in the dark, planless and ultimately unsatisfying. A sound psychodynamic training provides this basic understanding and it is this that I believe these young people are seeking. Thus their search represents a corrective swing of the pendulum away from the blind rejection of cognitive understanding that has characterized so many of the newer psychotherapies.

As I have said elsewhere (16), "the psychotherapeutic challenge of the future is to so improve our theoretical and diagnostic approaches to psychopathology as to be able to most knowledgeably and flexibly apply to each patient the particular treatment technique and the particular kind of therapist that together will most effectively achieve the desired therapeutic goal." To achieve such a goal we need more than just empathy and intuition; we also need to broaden and extend our psychodynamic knowledge and understanding. And so we come full circle, albeit in a somewhat different context, to Freud's perceptive statement: "The voice of the intellect is a soft one, but it does not rest until it has gained a hearing!"

REFERENCES

1. Quoted by Lewis, N. D. C. in Historical Roots of Psychotherapy, in Masserman, J. and Moreno, J. (Eds.): *Progress in Psychotherapy,* Vol. III, New York: Grune & Stratton, 1958, p. 25.
2. Freud, S.: *The Future of an Illusion.* London: The Hogarth Press, 1934, p. 93.
3. Freud, S.: *Ibid.,* p. 77.
4. Freud, S.: *New Introductory Lectures,* New York: W. W. Norton, 1933, p. 112.

5. Marmor, J.: Psychoanalysis and Psychiatric Practice, in Masserman, J. (Ed.): *Current Psychiatric Therapies,* Vol. IV, New York: Grune & Stratton, 1961, pp. 131-138.
6. Marmor, J.: Psychoanalytic Therapy as an Educational Process, in Masserman, J. (Ed.): *Science and Psychoanalysis,* Vol. V, New York: Grune & Stratton, 1962, pp. 286-299.
7. Marmor, J.: Psychoanalytic Therapy and Theories of Learning, in Masserman, J. (Ed.): *Science and Psychoanalysis,* Vol. VII, New York: Grune & Stratton, 1964, pp. 265-279.
8. Marmor, J.: The Nature of the Psychotherapeutic Process, in Usdin, G. L. (Ed.): *Psychoneurosis and Schizophrenia.* Philadelphia: Lippincott, 1966, pp. 66-75.
9. Wolpe, J.: *Psychotherapy by Reciprocal Inhibition.* Stanford: Stanford University Press, 1958.
10. Rogers, C.: *Client Centered Therapy.* Boston: Houghton Mifflin, 1951.
11. Roszack, T.: *The Making of the Counter Culture.* New York: Doubleday, 1969.
12. Lazarus, A. A.: *Behavior Therapy and Beyond.* New York: McGraw-Hill, 1971.
13. Brady, J. P.: Psychotherapy by a Combined Behavioral and Dynamic Approach, *Compr. Psychiatry,* 9:536-543, 1968.
14. Marks, I. M. and Gelder, M. G.: Common Ground Between Behavior Therapy and Psychodynamic Methods, *Brit. J. Med. Psychol.,* 39: 11-23, 1966.
15. Feather, B. W. and Rhoads, J. M.: Psychodynamic Behavior Therapy, *Arch. Gen. Psych.,* 26:503-511, 1972.
16. Marmor, J.: Dynamic Psychotherapy and Behavior Therapy, *Arch. Gen. Psych.,* 24:22-28, 1971.

6.

The Future of Medical Education and Its Implications for Psychiatry

JOHN P. HUBBARD, M.D.

and

BRYCE TEMPLETON, M.D.

This title, "The Future of Medical Education and Its Implications for Psychiatry," implies an assumption of clairvoyance that is far from realistic. We can gain some comfort, however, from the fact that the direction in which medical education appears to be heading has been the subject of intensive study by the National Board of Medical Examiners and an extraordinarily active and effective, specially appointed committee known as the Committee on Goals and Priorities. This committee is spoken of as the GAP Committee, an acronym very familiar to you and one which has a well-established ring of advance, of movement from where we are to where we may be going.

Our GAP Committee is a small group of 11 individuals carefully selected to make recommendations to the National

Board as to its responsibilities, its goals and priorities, in relation to the on-rushing tumultuous changes that are so evident in medical education throughout the United States today. For the past two years this committee has worked with impressive dedication, projecting a ten year forecast of medical education encompassing all phases of medical education from entry into the system throughout the physician's professional career. This forecast then provided the staging area for the formulation of recommendations for the evaluation system as it relates to medical education, certification for licensure, and certification for specialty practice. We cannot—or at least should not—anticipate the report of our committee. But neither can we refrain from mentioning some of the determining factors that our committee has been studying—factors that have important implications not only for the future of medical education in general, but also, specifically, for the field of psychiatry.

Turning to the forecast of medical education over the course of the next ten years, three important concepts have developed in the recent past that are bound to have profound implications for psychiatry. First is the position taken jointly by the Association of American Medical Colleges and the AMA Council on Medical Education redefining the essentials of medical education. The role of the medical school is described as preparation for further education in a graduate training program and not as preparation for the independent practice of medicine. This statement is so predictive of things to come that we would like to quote the following excerpt verbatim:

> The undergraduate period of medical education leading to the M.D. degree is no longer sufficient to prepare a

> student for independent medical practice without supplementation by a graduate training period which will vary in length depending upon the type of practice the student selects.

The statement then proceeds to comment upon the medical school curriculum during these years of preparation for further training:

> There is no single curriculum that can be prescribed for the undergraduate period of medical education. Each student should acquire a foundation of knowledge in the basic sciences that will permit the pursuit of any of the several careers that medicine offers. The student should be comfortably familiar with the methods and skills utilized in the practice of clinical medicine. Instructions should be sufficiently comprehensive so as to include the study of both mental and physical disease in patients who are hospitalized as well as ambulatory. At the same time, it should foster and encourage the development of the specific and unique interests of each student by tailoring the program in accordance with the student's preparation, competence, and interests.

A second, closely related concept that bears more on graduate medical education than on undergraduate medical education is the concept of corporate responsibility for the continuum of medical education. This concept first gained prominent attention within the medical education establishment when it appeared in the 1965 report of the AAMC, known as the Coggeshall Report (1). This report stated that "it is increasingly clear that the need of the future is for the university to assume comprehensive responsibility for medical education—extending to the pre-medical student, the medical student, the intern, the resident and the practicing physician."

A year later, 1966, the Report of the Citizens Commission on Graduate Medical Education, commissioned by the AMA and generally known as the Millis Report (2), similarly recommended that "each teaching hospital organize its staff, through an educational council, a committee on graduate medical education, or some similar means, so as to make its programs of graduate medical education a corporate responsibility rather than the individual responsibilities of particular medical or surgical services or heads of services." The concept of corporate responsibility for graduate medical education was then extended and formally accepted as follows by the AAMC at its Annual Meeting in October, 1971 (3):

> Graduate medical education ultimately should become a responsibility of academic medical centers ... Faculties of academic medical centers should develop, in conjunction with their parent universities and their teaching hospitals, programmatic plans for taking responsibility for graduate medical education in a manner analogous to presently established procedures for undergraduate medical education. Assumption of this responsibility by academic medical center faculties means that the entire faculty will establish mechanisms: to determine the general objectives and goals of its graduate programs and the nature of their teaching environment; to review curricula and instructional plans for each specific program; to arrange for evaluating graduate student programs periodically; and to confirm student readiness to sit for examinations by appropriate specialty boards.

The third interrelated concept that is changing and shaping medical education concerns the further recommendation of the Millis Report that, in looking toward the continuum of medical education, "the internship as a separate and distinct portion of medical education be abandoned and that the internship and residency years be combined into a single period of graduate medical education called a residency and planned as a unified whole (4)."

These three concepts have implications for the future of medical education in psychiatry, especially at the graduate level.

Implications for Specialty Training in Psychiatry

Psychiatry is only one of the specialties in which students are finding themselves up against career decisions earlier and earlier during the medical school years. Elective time during medical school may offer some opportunity for exploration of specialty tracks but the trend is away from this opportunity during an internship year. This trend is not without its critics. Among others, George Engel took a position in favor of an article appearing in *The New Physician* (5) that decried the "interment of the internship."

In addition to the movement toward abandoning the year of internship are pressures in the direction of shortening undergraduate medical education and residency training. For example, medical schools are being encouraged to design their curricula in such a fashion that most of the students will complete medical school in three years rather than the traditional four years. In all likelihood, this trend will preclude summer electives and the hard-to-define, sometimes disparaged, opportunity for maturation.

Now, therefore, with about one third of all U.S. medical schools on a three year curriculum, students in an increasing number of medical schools graduate after 32 to 36 months and go directly into residency training. Furthermore, with the flexibility and freedom of choice now available to students even in the three year curriculum, a student who is committed to a career in his chosen specialty—let us say psychiatry—can focus his interests and training in this specialized direction to the exclusion of a more rounded background in general medicine.

Beyond the medical school, with its redefined role of preparation for graduate medical education, the residency becomes the training ground for the practice of medicine. And it is in this phase of the continuum of medical education that problems of special importance for psychiatry appear along the road ahead. To the degree that corporate responsibility for graduate medical education may take hold, and to the degree, therefore, that residency programs become the responsibility of universities and their affiliated hospitals, the survival of residency programs in non-affiliated hospitals will be in jeopardy. Psychiatry will feel this influence rather more than other specialties. Of the 5,428 residency positions offered in psychiatry for the years 1972-73 (6), 1,480, about 27 percent, are in non-affiliated hospitals. This number of psychiatry residencies in non-affiliated hospitals is greater than that shown for any other specialty for the same reporting period and will bring about formidable problems if the move toward corporate responsibility for graduate medical education continues.

Further light is thrown on another feature of graduate education in psychiatry wherein this specialty stands out as quite different from all others. The statement is frequently made that virtually all who graduate from U.S. medical schools today enter specialty training. An examination of the extent of this trend was undertaken by our Committee on Goals and Priorities to serve as a guide for their deliberations related to specialty board certification. As a part of this study, a random sample of U.S. medical graduates for 1964 was analyzed according to self-designated specialty categories. For example, each individual in the sample who said he was a psychiatrist was so classified irrespective of whether he had been certified by the American Board of Psychiatry and Neurology. The same was done for all other specialties. With the help and cooperation of the specialty boards information was obtained to show how many of those who claimed specialty qualification had in fact had residencies in their specialties.

The results and implications of this study are being prepared for publication at an early date. In the meantime, however, some of the new data that appear to have particular importance for psychiatry is of much interest. Figure 1 deals with four of the major specialties: pediatrics, general surgery, internal medicine, and psychiatry and neurology. Here it is seen that 98 to 100 percent of those who said they were specialists in pediatrics, general surgery, or internal medicine had entered graduate training; for psychiatry and neurology 92 percent had entered graduate training. Similar percentages were found for other specialties; thus we have substantial evidence to support the universal trend toward graduate education.

LICENSURE AND SPECIALTY CERTIFICATION

The three concepts to which we alluded earlier (the unfinished nature of the pre-M.D. training, the emphasis upon corporate responsibility, and the need for coordination

%
100
80
60
40
20
0
100
99
98
92
Pediatrics
General Surgery
Internal Medicine
Psychiatry & Neurology
1964 GRADUATES
ENTERING GRADUATE MEDICAL EDUCATION

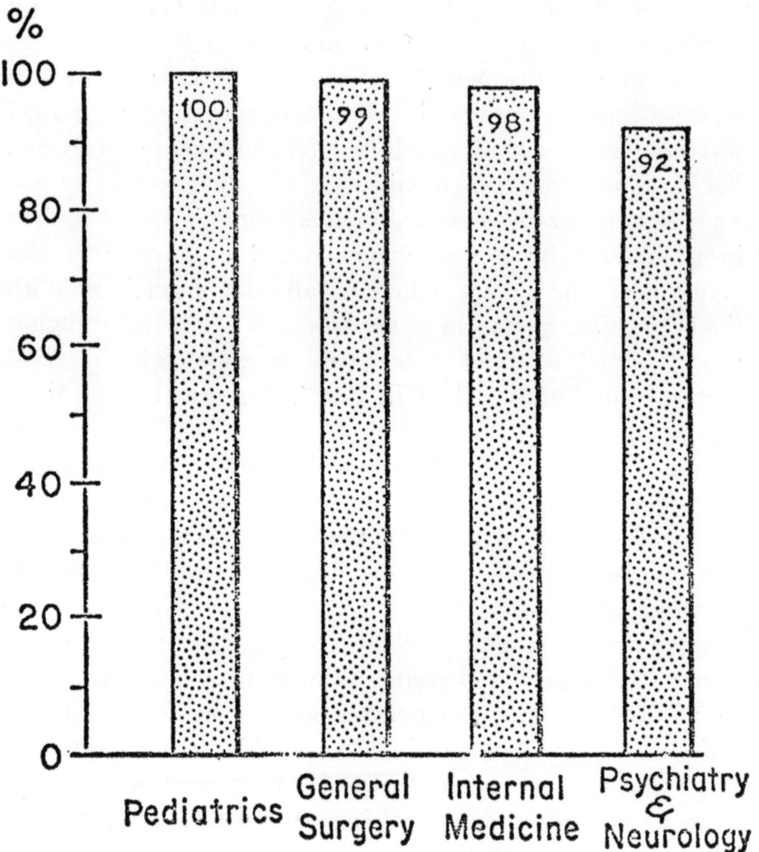

Figure 1

of an individual's post-M.D. training) also have significant implications for licensure and certification of those in the field of psychiatry.

Licensure has traditionally followed the completion of undergraduate medical education and the awarding of the M.D. degree—perhaps with a requirement of one additional year of graduate training known as the internship. Now, as we have seen, the role of the medical school is becoming redefined as preparation for graduate training, the free-standing year of internship is on the way out, and residency training is becoming a universal component of the continuum of medical education. The question is therefore being raised as to the reasonableness and justification of the granting of an unlimited license to practice medicine, surgery, or psychiatry at the midpoint of the continuum before the physician has had that period of supervised hospital experience that we know as the residency and that we consider essential to qualify an individual to assume responsibility for the care of patients. It seems likely that in the public interest official state board licensure will shift from the present midpoint in the continuum of medical education to a more logical and defensible point, signifying by certification that the physician has acquired the competence to provide patient care as an independent practitioner. Thus we may anticipate the day—perhaps not too far away—when qualification for a medical license will be related to specialty certification rather than to an all-encompassing certification upon completion of the undergraduate years of medical education.

The study of specialty training, referred to above, included a determination of the extent to which those who entered residency training undertook to obtain certification in that specialty, at least as far as taking the written examination of the specialty board. Thus we were looking for those who, having elected graduate education, had considered it important to meet the requirements of the American Board in their specialty. Figure 2 shows that for pediatrics, general surgery, and internal medicine, 80 to 90 percent of the sample

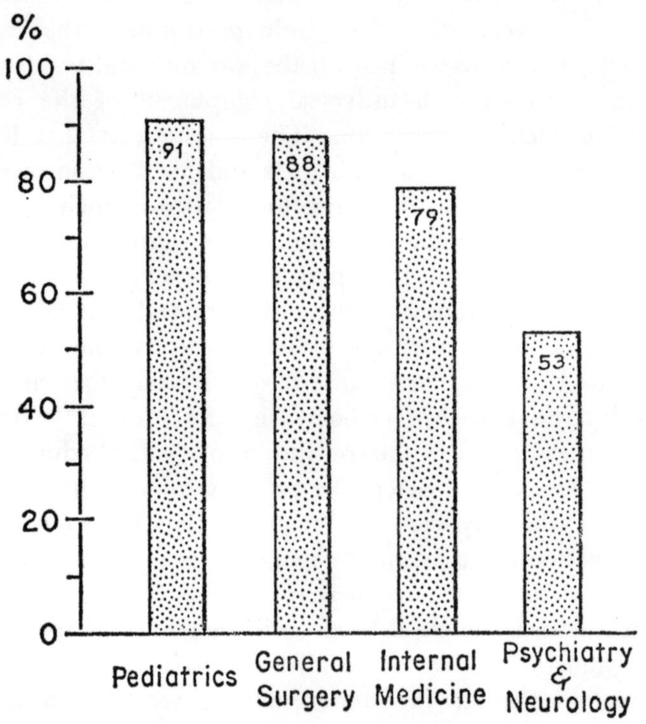

1964 GRADUATES
TAKING WRITTEN EXAMINATION OF SPECIALTY BOARD

Figure 2

of the 1964 graduates of the U.S. medical schools were candidates for certification. For psychiatry and neurology, however, only 53 percent ever appeared for the written examination of the American Board of Psychiatry and Neurology. The question might fairly be asked if, for some unknown reason, the graduating class of 1964 was in some way exceptional or out-of-step with annual statistics. A random sample of the graduating class of 1960 showed very similar results, as seen in Figure 3. For psychiatry and neurology, 58 percent of the sample of this class completed graduate education and signed up for the written examination of the specialty board as compared with 83 to 94 percent of those preparing for the other three specialty groups.

In a somewhat similar analysis, Taylor and Torrey reported that approximately one third of the nation's practicing psychiatrists have obtained specialty board certification (7). The difference between the Taylor and Torrey figures (approximately 33 percent) and our own (approximately 56 percent) probably reflects the different population studied. Taylor and Torrey apparently included graduates of foreign medical schools, whereas our own study focused exclusively on graduates of U.S. medical schools.

The motivations of individual physicians seeking specialty board certification vary. In addition to individual pride, certification usually brings tangible benefits including an increased likelihood of obtaining hospital appointments with admitting privileges, and increased income for those physicians in salaried positions in certain federal and state facilities.

The above figures indicating the number of psychiatrists who become certified must be viewed within the context of the large number of institutions that are in great need of

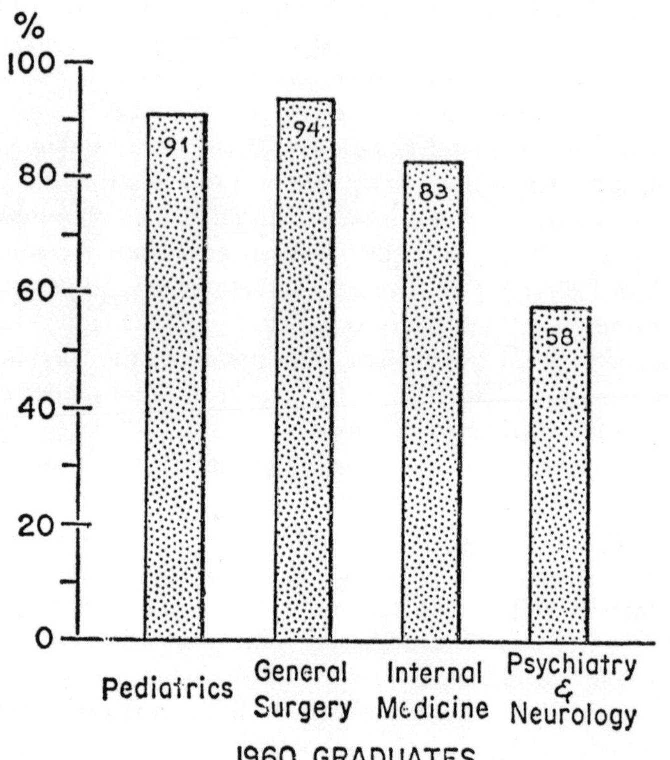

1960 GRADUATES
TAKING WRITTEN EXAMINATION OF SPECIALTY BOARD

Figure 3

psychiatric services and hire physicians who designate themselves as specialists in psychiatry on the basis of one or two years of graduate education. The possibility of improving one's chances of obtaining private hospital admitting privileges probably serves little use to the many psychiatrists whose private practices are based outside the hospital. Another factor that must be considered is the number of psychiatrists who first obtained training in general psychiatry and then obtained training in psychoanalysis, accepting membership in the American Psychoanalytic Association as final proof of their competence to practice (8).

In his response to the controversial article by Taylor and Torrey, mentioned above, Frazier has outlined some of the complexities of the certification procedures as viewed by the American Board (9). These complexities include the inevitable fragmentation of knowledge as practitioners develop subspecialty skills, and the difficulty of predicting the competencies that will be required 10-30 years after the psychiatrist becomes certified by the American Board. Frazier has also pointed to some of the steps which the American Board adopted in attempting to improve its certification procedure, including the formation of a long-range planning committee, the invitation of representatives of other specialty boards to observe the examination procedures, and the plans by several of the medical specialty boards to coordinate their research efforts in exploring new methods of assessing the competence of physicians.

Following successful completion of specialty board certification, young physicians have traditionally breathed an extra sigh of relief with the expectation that, barring some catastrophe, their license and specialty certification conferred a lifetime sanction to practice medicine. It is not surprising that this type of professional security is bowing to public insistence that doctors be required to demonstrate throughout the lifetime of their clinical work that they are maintaining professional competence (10).

The American Board of Family Practice was the first specialty board to respond to this need by requiring its diplomates to obtain recertification every six years. The first Family Practice Certificates issued in 1970 specify "good until 1976." Since this historic decision, two other specialty boards, the American Board of Internal Medicine and the American Board of Plastic Surgery, have also committed themselves to recertification, a trend which will surely gain momentum and spread to other specialties.

The rapid expansion of the medical self-assessment programs reflects an awareness by physicians of the need to assess the adequacy of their fund of medical knowledge. In spite of these voluntary efforts of many physicians and specialty societies, mandatory reassessment is highly likely. At this time we cannot predict what form recertification might take. Certainly we need some means of determining whether a physician has been updating his fund of knowledge. Also, we need a mechanism of assuring the public of the quality of care provided by each physician on a day-to-day basis. Efforts are underway now to explore the use of the medical chart audit as a means of assessing the individual physician's performance. Determining standards of care which can be applied fairly will be a challenge in non-psychiatric clinical fields as well as in psychiatry. Is there a realistic technique that will provide a valid and reasonably economical measure of the day-to-day quality of a psychiatrist's outpatient practice? As yet, the question is unanswered.

THE CONTRIBUTION OF EDUCATIONAL SCIENCES

Historically the National Board has derived great value from the educational sciences outside the field of medicine. This was exemplified in the 1950s by our collaboration with the Educational Testing Service whereby we were able to adapt to medical subject matter the techniques of highly reliable multiple-choice examinations (11). In the 1960s, in collaboration with the American Institute of Research, we utilized the critical incident technique to define the competencies expected of young physicians at the internship level of training (12).

Current developments within the educational sciences have implications for training in psychiatry at both the undergraduate (the pre-M.D.) and graduate level. In all likelihood, the planners of the 1967 Conference on Psychiatry in Medical Education held similar values, as evidenced by their invitation to Ralph Tyler to deliver the opening charge to the participants (13). Dr. Tyler's charge focused on three important areas which are still relevant in planning the future of psychiatric education: the formulation of educational objectives, the development of learning experiences, and the development of improved means of appraising student progress.

FORMULATION OF EDUCATIONAL OBJECTIVES

The increasing interest among educators in specifying educational objectives has already begun to have a major impact on professional training (14,15). A number of medical school departments, in some instances entire medical schools, are going through the struggle of defining more precisely their educational objectives. Whether or not each department of psychiatry should determine its own set of objectives remains unanswered. Although the faculty may derive some special heuristic benefits, the costs in terms of faculty time are high. Requiring every department of psychiatry to formulate independently its own set of objectives seems as unrealistic as to require every department to produce its own textbook in psychiatry. In all likelihood, some national coordination of effort would conserve faculty time and would create a better set of objectives with broader applicability than could possibly be achieved by any single psychiatry department working independently.

On what basis will the objectives for psychiatry be established? If the overall purpose of the medical curriculum is to produce competent physicians, then the specification of objectives must be based on careful documentation of the necessary competencies,—i.e., the knowledge, attitudes, and the interpersonal and motor skills which will permit each physician to provide good medical care. The available role-defining techniques that permit some systematic collection of data about the required competencies include the critical incident technique, task analysis inventories, and direct observation. As noted above, in 1966 the National Board utilized the critical incident technique to define the competencies required of the intern. More recently the National Board has utilized the task inventory approach in defining the competencies of the assistant to the primary care physician. In order to develop a meaningful itemization of educational objectives in psychiatry, one of the above approaches would help to answer the following questions: (1) What psychiatric knowledge and skills should be required of the medical student before granting him the M.D. degree and the right to take on responsibility, under supervision, for patient care? (2) Are there any differences in the type and amount of psychiatric knowledge and skills that should be required of the student who plans a career in psychiatry in comparison with the psychiatric knowledge and skills required of the student planning a career in some other clinical discipline? and (3) What psychiatric knowledge and skills should be required of every psychiatric resident before he is certified as competent to assume responsibility for independent practice? The answers to these questions itemized in terms of measurable behaviors will be important in planning the learning experiences of students and residents.

DEVELOPMENT OF LEARNING EXPERIENCES

A number of developments suggest that the next decade will bring a major growth in the availability of self-instructional materials for medical students and residents. The advantages of self-instructional material include the following: (1) the student can proceed at a pace consistent with his own learning abilities; (2) he can go over the material as often as necessary until he has mastered it; and (3) the design of the materials frequently facilitates the inclusion of mechanisms to provide each student with frequent feedback concerning his achievement.

Although programmed texts have been widely used in other fields, relatively few psychiatrists have attempted to utilize this technique in developing texts in psychiatry (16,17,18). However, psychiatrists have done well in exploring the value of certain technological innovations which have shown promise of being particularly suited to the teaching of interviewing and communication skills. The use of tape recorders, one-way mirrors, and more recently, the videotape recorder have all been well documented.

Each year brings the availability of an increasing number of new products having attributes which will be especially useful in the design of self-instructional units. Some products that have become available only recently include portable cassette recorders, synchronized sound film strip projectors, inexpensive video-recorders, and computer programs involving natural language interaction between student and instructor. These learning modalities will all have important implications for psychiatric training.

Our comments about the need for nationwide cooperative planning and development in the specification of educational objectives are equally applicable to self-instructional materials in psychiatry. Successful development of technology-assisted instruction will require the same degree of planning and effort currently carried out by groups of authors and editors who assemble some of our prestigious texts in psychiatry and other medical fields. This type of effort will be essential if we are to produce material that will be of sufficient quality for use by students at a large number of medical schools. Groups with special interest in developing these methods would do well to review educational journals concerned with media technology (for example, the *Journal of Educational Technology*).

Innovations in the development of computer and human simulations already show promise of providing us with new dimensions for techniques in training. Harless's Computer-Assisted Simulation of the Clinical Encounter (CASE) provides students with a variety of experiences in diagnostic problem-solving (19). In these simulations, the student takes the role of the physician and the computer takes the role of a specific patient with a specific medical and psychosocial history and abnormal physical and laboratory findings. This system provides the student with (1) greater exposure to a planned variety of clinical problems; (2) an opportunity to practice and repractice data gathering and diagnostic skills in a setting in which errors do not adversely affect the patient; and (3) early feedback about performance as viewed, not by a single instructor, but by a consensus of experts in the field.

A small but progressively expanding library of these CASE simulations is available through the Lister Hill National Center for Biomedical Communications for students in medical schools that have appropriate computer terminal facilities.

One of the simulations available through the Lister Hill Center (a case identified by the name of Ester McGrory) represents an attempt to incorporate the teaching of certain objectives in psychiatry with certain objectives from other clinical disciplines (20). In this particular simulation, the student is required to characterize the nature of a psychological crisis in a patient who develops congestive heart failure following a long history of rheumatic valvular heart disease.

This form of computer-assisted instruction will probably have an increasing impact on a large number of medical students. The library contains more than a dozen simulations. Therefore, it will be important to avoid dwelling on the limitations of these simulations. Instead we should review our educational objectives carefully to determine which of these objectives are especially suited to this new educational tool and also to decide what role psychiatrists should play in the design of these simulations. For example, should these simulated patients demonstrate a logically consistent personality? How extensive should the psychosocial data base be about each patient? How much psychosocial information should the student be encouraged or required to obtain in each medical or surgical simulation? Do any of the simulations include clinical problems of a primarily psychiatric nature? How often do the planning and management decisions depend upon having obtained some of the psychosocial data?

Barrows and Abrahamson were the first to publish an account describing the utilization of actors programmed to adopt a specific clinical history and physical examination findings as a means of providing students with an opportunity to practice certain clinical skills (21). This simulated patient technique is under study by a number of schools to determine its usefulness as an instructional method (22).

With advances in technology-assisted instruction, the role of the teacher will continue to change substantially (23). No longer a "talk and chalk" person, a major segment of his time and energies will be occupied with the management of educational resources: planning educational programs, organizing and implementing the curriculum, staying abreast of national activities, participating in the national development of and sharing of instructional materials, and designing and implementing the intramural evaluation program (24). In order to facilitate effective performance in this new role, the teacher will find it increasingly advantageous to obtain some formal training in the educational sciences.

Although we have predicted major growth in self-instructional materials, medical students and residents will continue to need personal contact with members of the faculty by means of small group activities. This personal contact will continue to be an important source of inspiration and encouragement for trainees.

EVALUATION OF INDIVIDUAL COMPETENCE

Any effective evaluation technique must be reliable (i.e., provide reproducible measurements) and valid (i.e., measure what it was designed to measure). In addition, the administration of the evaluation technique must be feasible from the point of view of costs, the number of candidates to be tested, and other logistical considerations.

Of the available evaluation techniques, multiple-choice testing has evolved into a highly reliable technique of assessing an examinee's fund of knowledge. Although we expect that this approach will continue to serve in a useful fashion, further refinements can be expected, For example, several groups have experimented with computer presentations of multiple-choice test items; the correctness of an examinee's responses influences the subsequent selection of multiple-choice items displayed by the computer so that a more rapid assessment of an individual's overall achievement level can be determined (25).

The use of film material in conjunction with multiple-choice examinations focusing on an interview between a physician and a patient or some other aspect of clinical behavior may offer important additional dimensions in assessing an examinee's observational skills or knowledge of the appropriate verbal interventions. In our experience film examinations have been costly to produce and administer on a national basis. On occasion we have informally reviewed film examinations used by individual medical schools. These reviews have been hampered because the departments using the film examinations have only infrequently assembled item statistics describing the student performance on each test item. Moreover, in a number of instances, many of the test items do not actually require observation of a film. Miller's Systems Analysis Index for Diagnosis (SAID), originally designed as a means of providing a more reliable method of making a psychiatric assessment of a patient suspected of having a psychiatric problem, may prove useful, in a modified form, as the basis of a film examination (26).

Considerable caution should be exercised in concluding that scores on a film examination will predict overall interviewing abilities. One recent report described a slight negative correlation between the results of a film examination assessing the knowledge of the correct usage of interviewing principles, and the results of assessments of student interviewing skills made on the basis of directly observing the examinees (27).

Many psychiatrists are familiar with the patient management problem (PMP) technique utilized in the 1969 and 1972 American Psychiatric Association self-assessment programs. With this technique the examinee obtains data and makes management decisions by means of an eraser or felt-pen. With each action taken, the examinee obtains information concerning the action taken. This technique has worked especially well in the assessment of an examinee's ability to interpret the significance of history and physical examination findings and to make appropriate use of the laboratory. Recently we have been exploring the use of the PMP technique to generate hypotheses and obtain additional data about a patient's psychological state. Although this technique would appear to be useful in assessing a number of educational objectives relevant to psychiatry, considerable additional work will be required to ascertain the reliability and validity of this approach.

For the past several years the National Board of Medical Examiners and the American Board of Internal Medicine have been jointly exploring the use of a computerized simulation of the physician-patient encounter known as the computer-based examination (CBX). Recently the CBX program has included the use of the CASE simulation. Although these studies are currently oriented toward internal medicine, the results will have important implications for evaluation of professional competence in other specialties, including psychiatry. Computer simulations appear to provide a means of assessing certain history-taking skills and the examinee's ability to generate and reject, in an appropriate fashion, diagnostic hypotheses. The history-taking portion of this new evaluation procedure will probably require validation by comparing performance on this portion of the simulation with performance of interviewing skills as measured by direct observation.

The assessment of interviewing skills by directly observing students interviewing simulated patients is currently under investigation by several groups (28). The use of *interaction analysis* to describe the interview process and the use of check lists to quantitate the amount of appropriate data obtained by the examinee show promise of providing us with fairly reliable estimates of an examinee's interviewing and interpersonal skills. The National Board is currently beginning exploration of methods to assess interpersonal skills, but it is much too early to say if and in what form this assessment might take place.

Although a medical student or house officer may possess the requisite knowledge and skills to provide medical care in a satisfactory fashion, his possession of this knowledge and these skills does not necessarily insure that he will perform satisfactorily on a day-by-day basis. We need additional techniques that will permit us to assess the day-to-day performance of trainees. Two approaches that may be especially useful to departments of psychiatry include audits of audiotape recordings of physician-patient contacts and audits of the trainees' entries in the medical chart (29).

The availability of audiotape cassette recorders provides a means of having students and house officers record all of their patient contacts, a small segment of which can be subsequently selected on a random basis and reviewed in either a group or individual supervisory session. In order to reduce costs, the recorder could be shared by two trainees who alternate the use of it on a weekly or biweekly basis. The tapes can be erased following supervisory sessions and then made available for reuse.

Although medical teachers have been reviewing charts for many years, a medical chart audit represents an attempt to define in a collaborative way what is required in the chart. As far as medical students are concerned, this might focus primarily on the charting process itself in terms of the completeness and accuracy of the data base entered. An audit may also assess the extent to which management decisions carried out by residents measure up to the standards set by a faculty committee.

Summary

Several concepts will have important implications for training in psychiatry and the licensure and certification of psychiatrists. These concepts include the unfinished nature of pre-M.D. training, and the need for universities to assume responsibility for the continuum of medical education. These concepts will have a major impact on psychiatric training especially at the graduate level. In addition, the rapid advances in the educational sciences will bring with them major changes at all levels of medical education with improvement in our ability to specify educational objectives, a movement toward national coordination of the development of self-instructional materials, and improvements in our evaluation techniques. Furthermore, the role of the faculty member will continue to change from that of classroom lecturer to one of a manager of educational resources.

In pointing to some of the observable tides of medical education and their implications for psychiatry, we have been raising more questions than answers. This was our intention, for in so doing we would like to point to the need for information—more, much more, factual data that can serve to guide the specialty of psychiatry as it faces up to the challenges that arise from within the educational system and from society. Psychiatry needs broad studies to provide the groundwork from which the objectives can be defined, in measurable terms, at the undergraduate and graduate levels of training. These studies will need to include information about manpower utilization, the extent and lack of certification, and the extent to which the individual psychiatrist is maintaining his professional competence.

REFERENCES

1. Coggeshall, Lowell T.: *Planning for Medical Progress through Education.* Evanston, Illinois: Association of American Medical Colleges, 1965.
2. *The Graduate Education of Physicians,* the Report of the Citizens Commission on Graduate Medical Education. Chicago: American Medical Association, 1966, pp. 60-61.
3. *Bulletin of the Association of American Medical Colleges,* vol. VI, No. 9, Nov. 15, 1971.
4. *The Graduate Education of Physicians,* op. cit., p. 62.
5. Engel, George L.: Letter to the Editor, *The New Physician,* March, 1972, p. 126.

6. *Directory of Approved Internships and Residencies.* Chicago: American Medical Association, 1972.
7. Taylor, R. L. and Torrey, E. F.: The Pseudo-regulation of American Psychiatry. *Amer. J. Psychiat.,* 129:658-663, 1972.
8. Rogow, A. A.: *The Psychiatrists.* New York: Dell Publishing Co., 1970.
9. Frazier, S. H.: A Commentary on "The Pseudo-regulation of American Psychiatry." *Amer. J. Psychiat.,* 129:664-668, 1972.
10. U.S. Dept. of Health, Education, and Welfare, *Report on Licensure and Related Health Personnel Credentialing,* June 1971.
11. Hubbard, John P.: *Measuring Medical Education: The Tests and Test Procedures of the National Board of Medical Examiners.* Philadelphia: Lea & Febiger, 1971.
12. Hubbard, John P., et al.: An Objective Evaluation of Clinical Competence. *New Eng. J. Med.,* 272:1321-1328, 1965.
13. Early, L. W., et al.: *Teaching Psychiatry in Medical School.* Washington, D. C.: American Psychiatric Association, 1969.
14. Bacchus, H.: Programming Educational Objectives in Internal Medicine. *J. Med. Educ.,* 47:708-711, 1972.
15. Baker, Frank B.: Computer-based Instructional Management Systems: A First Look. *Rev. Educ. Res.,* 41:51-70, 1971.
16. Beckett, Peter G. S., et al.: *A Teaching Program in Psychiatry, Vol. II: Psychoneurosis, Organic Brain Disease, Psychopharmacology.* Detroit: Wayne State Press, 1969.
17. Froelich, R. E. and Bishop, F. Marion: *Medical Interviewing, A Programmed Manual.* St. Louis, Mo.: C. V. Mosby Co., 1969.
18. Mathis, J. L., et al.: *Basic Psychiatry, a Primer of Concept and Terminology.* New York: Appleton-Century-Croft, 1968.
19. Harless, W. G., et al.: CASE: A Computer Assisted Simulation of the Clinical Encounter. *J. Med. Educ.,* 46:443-448, 1971.
20. Harless, W. G. and Templeton, B.: The Potential of CASE for Evaluating Undergraduate Psychiatric Education. Presented at the NIMH Congress on Evaluation of Undergraduate Psychiatry, June 22-23, 1972.
21. Barrows, H. S. and Abrahamson, S.: The Programmed Patient: A Technique for Assessing Student Performance in Clinical Neurology. *J. Med. Educ.,* 39:802-805, 1964.
22. Helfer, R. and Hess, J.: An Experimental Model for Making Objective Measurements of Interviewing Skills. *J. Clin. Psych.,* 26:327-331, 1970.
23. Lomax, D. E.: A Review of British Research in Teacher Education. *Rev. of Educ. Res.,* 42:289-326, 1972.
24. Mager, R. F. and Beach, K. M., Jr.: *Developing Vocational Instruction.* Belmont, Calif.: Fearon Publishers, 1967.
25. Woods, Elinor M.: Recent Application of Computer Technology to School Testing Programs. *Rev. of Educ. Res.,* 40:525-540, 1970.
26. Miller, P. R.: *SAID Handbook, Systems Analysis Index of Basic Psychiatric Syndromes.* Paul R. Miller, Davis, Calif., 1972.

27. Ware, J. E., et al.: A Negative Relationship between Understanding Interviewing Principles and Interview Performance. *J. Med. Educ.,* 46: 620-622, 1971.
28. Helfer, R. E.: An Objective Comparison of the Pediatric Interviewing Skills of Freshmen and Senior Medical Students. *Ped.,* 45:623-627, 1970.
29. Templeton, B.: Evaluating Student Performance, in D. G. Langsley, et al. (Eds.): *Mental Health in the New Medical Schools.* San Francisco: Jossey-Bass, Inc., 1973.

7.

Resistances to Innovation in Psychiatric Training as Exemplified by Marital Therapy

PETER A. MARTIN, M.D.

and

HAROLD I. LIEF, M.D.

INTRODUCTION

Both authors have been teaching psychiatric residents for many years. We have also devoted much of our professional lives to the treatment of marital problems. Curious about the extent of training in marital therapy, as well as in family therapy, we surveyed university based psychiatric training programs in the United States. We anticipated and found significant resistances to these newer modalities of therapy. In turn, this led to an attempt to delineate and describe the factors underlying the resistances to change in training.

We approach this problem with two conflicting biases. One is our firm belief that marital and family therapy are two of the most important methods of treatment available to the psychiatrist and ought to be part of his clinical skills and, therefore, should be included in his training. A second bias is that the enormous increase in demand by society for a vast array of services has created great strain on residency programs and has accounted for the tendency to develop an "uncritical ecleticism" (1) and for psychiatry to ride "madly in all directions (2). Ornstein (3) has pointed out the need to develop a core curriculum based on "skills, attitudes and fundamental knowledge that *remain common to all forms of psychiatric endeavor.*" If resistance to innovative modalities were based rationally on the need to define and develop such a core curriculum, one would anticipate that marital and family therapy would *at least* be available as electives. Much of the resistance, however, is based on a failure to understand the importance or the nature of these forms of treatment, or on an avoidance of them because of the absence of teachers skilled in these areas, or on even less rational reasons. Clearly, similar resistances to other innovations in psychiatric training take place in a similar fashion. Bringing them out into the open for discussion may lead to several solutions, one of which is suggested at the end of the paper.

RESISTANCE TO CHANGE

Resistances to innovation in psychiatric training may be caused by a variety of factors: faculty may be unimpressed with the possible changes; change may threaten the status of departmental decision makers; skills in implementing change, e.g., skillful teachers of a new therapeutic modality, may be deficient; other areas competing for attention may win out; economic factors may play a role; residents may resist adding to their workload, because of the fear of additional service demands, or balk at the demand of additional reading, or shy away from the emotional burdens created by unfamiliar therapeutic situations. Over and above these rational or semi-rational causes of resistance to change in psychiatric training, however, are resistances created by prejudice and plain inertia.

Although a few psychiatric training programs are in the process of continual change, some to such an extent that a third-year resident is unable to help a first-year resident anticipate his program with any degree of certitude, many more are so hidebound by inertia (the resistance to change itself rather than the fear of the consequences of change) that they continue to carry out their training in the same way year after year, almost oblivious of the changes in the field. As one despairing younger faculty member remarked, "it would be easier to move a graveyard." Often enough, inertia is rationalized by bias—"our way is proven to be more effective"; a "psychiatrist does not need to know that—a social worker or a psychiatric nurse or an aide can do that," etc. It is not surprising to students of the human condition to see how often the need for status and privilege is hidden by protective prejudices.

In this paper the authors attempt to explore, albeit in a rather simplistic fashion, some of the factors playing a part in the resistances to change in psychiatric training, using marital therapy as the example of possible change. It would be possible, of course, to study the factors in change by studying some other possible innovations in training such as having the in-patient service training after the first year rather than in its traditional first year slot, or training in the team concept in the delivery of mental health care, or training in what is loosely called "medical psychology," bypassing some non-essential aspects of medical training for a potential psychotherapist. (One could even study the psychosocial factors in *failing to resist change* as in the case of the bandwagon reaction to the idea of community health centers.) We chose marital therapy because both authors are deeply committed to this form of therapy and teach it in their respective institutions and because, in our view, there is a great need for this form of treatment in practice while, at the same time, until recently there seemed to be relatively little interest in teaching marital therapy to psychiatric residents. To us, the contrast between demand for therapy by couples in distress and the apparent failure to train residents to meet this demand is striking; it was this contrast that led to the study we are reporting.

NEED FOR MARITAL THERAPY

The evidence that there is great demand for services is based on the increasing request for marital therapy in specialized clinics such as the Marriage Council of Philadelphia, on the reports of psychiatrists in private practice who devote some of their time to this form of treatment, and on specific investigation of the frequency of marital problems in practice.

The Joint Commission on Mental Illness and Mental Health publication *Americans View Their Mental Health* (4) reported that marriage was the most important problem area in causing people to seek professional help. Forty-two percent of the people gave marriage and difficulties with the spouse as the major reason. Next were problems with children (12%) and other family relationships (5%). This means that 59% of people seek help because of marital or other family problems. Gurin, Veroff, and Feld also examined the relationship of the source of help used to the problem area and reported that 35% of a psychiatrist's practice was devoted to people who came because of marital problems; another 24% were people who came for help with other family relationship.

In a survey of a group of psychoanalysts, Sager, *et al.* (5) reported that marital difficulties prompted half the patients to seek treatment, and the existence of a major marital problem was uncovered in half of the remaining 50%. If this is a primary or major contributing factor in mental and emotional distress in from 59% to 75% of our patients in outpatient practice, why are the specific techniques needed in marital therapy, especially conjoint marital therapy, not taught more regularly and thoroughly in our training centers? How much are psychiatric teachers influenced by the dyadic model, buttressed by Freud's warnings against diluting the transference by seeing family members?

The same factors, though perhaps to a lesser degree, are at play in incorporating family therapy into training programs. As far back as 1954, the Group for the Advancement of Psychiatry in its report "Integration and Conflict in Family Behavior" (6) stated that a dramatic shift had taken place in American psychiatry. Whereas, formerly a psychiatrist could not afford to consider the family, now he could not afford to neglect the family. To what extent did this flat statement influence our training programs and to what extent was it unheard or resisted?

In carrying out this investigation, which involves a survey of university psychiatric training centers in the United States, we thus asked about family therapy as well as marital therapy.

Both fields are like fraternal twins—born within the same decade, they are about at the same stage of development. Olson (7) states: "they were both born and nurtured by interdisciplinary parentage and they have developed along separate but parallel lines. Like the development of an individual within the family unit, professions in their infancy need to learn from older and related disciplines so that some of the mistakes and pitfalls encountered by the older disciplines can be avoided or at least minimized once they are encountered."

Without firsthand experience in treating families or couples, it is difficult to comprehend the nature of the treatment process. The process itself is determined not only by the transactional dynamics of the people involved and the nature of the problems dealt with, but also by the approach of the therapist or therapists in the case of co-therapy. Therapy may be reality-oriented counseling or may be analytically-derived efforts at intrapsychic change in a group setting. Most of the time, however, the goal of therapeutic intervention is the modification of the transactions between husband and wife or among family members. It often allows for a combination of new insights into processes of perception and communication together with behavioral modifications of maladaptative behavior patterns, giving great play to the creative capacities of the therapist. It is a different ball game from one-to-one therapy and different skills are required. One is not a skilled family or marital therapist merely by virtue of becoming board eligible or certified in psychiatry. It does require specialized training.

(To make intelligible these forms of treatment to the uninitiated is impossible within the confines of this paper. The theoretical basis, or rationale, as well as the more specific skills and techniques can be found in the rather voluminous literature. The striking feature of these methods of treatment is the interplay between intrapsychic mechanisms and interpersonal behavior patterns. The transactional systems have to be understood and manipulated while the therapist is mindful of the drives, conflicts, inhibitions and symptoms of each participant. While it is complicated, it is also more exciting and intellectually and emotionally challenging than is dyadic therapy.)

METHOD

Each of the authors had independently thought of surveying departments of psychiatry in order to ascertain the extent of training in marital and family therapy. When Martin approached Lief about the possibility of doing this jointly, he discovered that Lief had already distributed a simple one-page questionnaire. A second, somewhat more detailed survey instrument was then mailed out. The results are a combination of the data derived from the returns to both questionnaires.

The first survey, an 80% return, demonstrated that only half the medical schools in the United States taught marital therapy in an organized fashion, and the range was from the single demonstration to six months of half-time supervised training. The other schools reporting claimed that they were teaching marital therapy but that it was informal and generally part of family therapy or of outpatient supervision. Clearly this was happenstance and a matter of luck in finding the couple to treat and an interested supervisor, and many residents in these programs would either have no training at all or very inadequate training.

A somewhat better situation for family therapy prevailed. Seventy-five percent of the schools reported formal training in family therapy. It was clear, however, that three-fourths of the 50% of schools reporting formal training in marital therapy taught it as part of family therapy. This means that few schools, perhaps 12 to 15%, are giving any emphasis to marital therapy as a distinct area for training and to the specialized skills required in marital therapy.

The second survey was organized to test five main assumptions: (1) a minority of training programs include definitive courses and supervision in marital therapy; (2) at those centers where specialized training in marital therapy occurs, it is often the result of a special interest in the area of one of the faculty members; (3) there is often a failure to "institutionalize" the teaching of marital therapy, so that if the faculty member with a special interest were to leave, training and interest in marital therapy would wane; (4) in those centers where teaching is based on the gifts and interests of a particular teacher rather than on a tradition of teaching marital therapy, a substantial number of residents tend to avoid opportunities for training even when available; (5) trainees in other mental health disciplines, by contrast, show a marked and increasing interest in training in marital therapy.

Questionnaires were distributed to chairmen of departments of psychiatry and to five residents at each training center. Fifty-eight training centers and 138 residents responded; Of the 58 centers, five still had no residency programs and were eliminated from the analysis of data.

The first three questions of the survey instrument were directed toward whether and how marital therapy was taught. Table 1 sumarizes this data.

TABLE 1

How Marital Therapy Is Taught

	*N**	% (rounded off)
As separate program	14	26
As part of:		
family therapy	24	45
outpatient therapy	14	26
sex therapy	1	—

* N=53 (52% response)

Every training center claimed it taught marital therapy, but only one in four taught it as a separate discipline, almost half as part of family therapy and one in four as part of the regular outpatient supervision. We have no data about the quality of these latter programs but can estimate with considerable assurance that it is often more of a promise than an actuality and that when it is taught at all, it is superficial and casual rather than sophisticated and serious.

The next several questions were directed toward the issue of whether training in marital and family therapy was the result of a special interest of a particular faculty member, whether these areas were regarded as part of the core curriculum, and if the faculty member with the special interest were to depart would the training continue. Table 2 summarizes this information.

It is clear that family therapy is part of the core curriculum in a higher number of training centers than is marital therapy and is now part of the teaching tradition in twice as many. Despite this, the fact that marital therapy is part of the core curriculum in two-thirds of the centers is very encouraging to those of us who regard this form of treatment

TABLE 2

"Institutionalized" Marital and Family Therapy

	Marital Therapy		*Family Therapy*	
	*N**	*%*	*N*	*%*
Core Curriculum	35	66	47	89
"Institutionalized"	16	30	34	64

* N=53

as an essential part of the therapeutic armamentarium of the psychiatrist.

In keeping with the greater emphasis on family therapy, 82% of the training programs included supervision in family therapy in contrast to the 68% which included supervision in marital therapy.

Twenty-four schools responded to our question aimed at discovering the reasons for failing to institutionalize marital and family therapy. The results are tabulated in Table 3. The three leading reasons are overlapping and interdigitating. It is somewhat astonishing to find that 10 schools still regard these fields as unimportant, but somewhat more un-

TABLE 3

Reasons for Failing to Institutionalize Marital and Family Therapy*

	*N***	*%*
Faculty Resistance	14	58
Unimportant Fields	10	42
Of No Value to Residents	6	25

* Multiple Responses Permitted
** N=24

TABLE 4

Reasons for Resistance of Residents as Reported by Faculty*

	N**	%
Avoidance of Overload	13	65%
Belief in Superficiality of these forms of treatment	7	35%
Fear of criticism for mistakes	7	35%
Biological psychiatry (5) and community psychiatry (2) more important	7	35%

* Multiple Responses Permitted
** N=20

derstandable that some regard them as of no value to residents, probably because they continue to think of them as the province of the psychologist, social worker or clergyman.

Other reasons for failing to institutionalize these forms of therapy are: they are dependent on the special interest, ability and enthusiasm of specific staff members; they represent an overload on the resources of faculty; because of shortage of staff there is a lack of familiarity with these fields among the faculty; these areas are considered anti-analytic and, hence, anti-dyadic, there is too much competition from other areas deemed more important; the curriculum is entirely dependent on the interest of the chairman.

Almost 40% of the programs report that residents have some resistances to training in these areas, even when training opportunities are available. Reasons for this resistance, as seen through the eyes of the departmental chairmen or the training program directors, are given in Table 4. Sixty-five

TABLE 5

Residents' Experience with Marital and Family Therapy

	Marital Therapy *% Yes*	*Family Therapy* *% Yes*
Didactic Course	25 (N=123)	32 (N=117)
Supervision	46 (N=123)	46 (N=117)
Special Interest of Faculty Member	56 (N=70)	58 (N=80)
Institutionalized	40 (N=62)	46 (N=69)

percent of the respondents felt that it was adding too much to an already overloaded curriculum; 35% felt that psychoanalysis was needed to bring about intrapsychic changes and the approaches of marital and family therapy were too superficial to be of therapeutic benefit. An equal number were said to be afraid of making mistakes in unfamiliar therapeutic terrain or considered other modalities more important.

SURVEY OF RESIDENTS

One hundred thirty-eight residents replied, of whom 15 were in the first year, 46 in the second, 59 in the third, 16 in the fourth, and 2 in the fifth. Review of the responses of the first-year residents made it clear that they had not had enough exposure to the variety of therapies to justify including them. This left 123 replies to be analyzed in Table 5. Twenty-five percent said they had received didactic training in marital therapy, a figure which matches the chairmen's report cited earlier (separate programs almost always involved didactic work such as lectures or seminars in addition to supervision). A somewhat higher percentage (32%) of residents reported receiving didactic courses in family

TABLE 6

Resistances of Residents to Marital and Family Therapy*

Item	*Weighted Score*
Overload (Emotional, Cognitive)	173 (N=96)
Not Important Areas	58 (N=43)
Dyadic Therapy is Only Effective Kind	57 (N=44)
Fear of Exposure to Criticism	50 (N=34)

* Two Choices Permitted in Rank Order

therapy. Forty-six percent of the residents reported receiving supervision in both marital and family therapy, indicating that some programs that had no didactic work did include supervision. Of the 70 residents who responded to a query regarding the influence of a particular faculty member, 56% felt that this was an important factor in establishing the training in marital therapy and almost the same percentage said the same about family therapy. The low number of respondents indicates that a substantial number of residents had no opinion about this factor. Only half of them had an opinion about whether the training would be continued if the faculty member were to depart and the results indicate that less than half felt that either marital therapy or family therapy would be continued if the interested faculty member left the department.

The survey responses revealed that 64% of the residents had taken advantage of the opportunity to participate in marital and family therapy training; almost 100% of the residents who failed to do so believed that such training should be available. Despite this, some residents resisted participation in these areas as revealed in Table 6. Using a technique of a weighted score for the two rank-ordered choices permitted, the analysis reveals that the most important factor, by a ratio of three to one, was the fear of overload, either emotional or cognitive. Their already crowded schedule made these areas appear to be a threat to their capacities to cope with additional material and demands. Other reasons checked off were that these were not important areas, or that dyadic therapy is the only effective kind, or that this would render the resident vulnerable to criticism from faculty. Some residents reported that they just feel more comfortable dealing with an individual person, others that their departments were moving away from patient care to consultation theory building and research, while some commented that these areas were the province of a social worker, and there was, in general, a lack of appeal because a structured theory that undergirds these fields does not exist. Among the unconscious determinants observed by the authors but not obtainable by a check list survey is the resistance created by the desire to avoid introspection concerning either their parents' marriage or their own marriage. This is almost always a factor in the training of marital therapists and accounts for the need to have sufficient time to work through the painful confrontation created by the need to more realistically examine one's own family relationships.

The residents were also asked why the department does not offer sufficient training in these areas. Some of the responses were: "There is a classical analytic bias in this department which does not include systems analysis required for dealing with systems larger than the dyad." "The staff here is overloaded. The faculty have not kept up. They are overwhelmed with the amount of work." "The more intensive desire for residents for supervision, the less time our faculty has for private patients. A complementary relationship is formed between resident and staff. The residents do not ask for supervision because it means greater exposure and the staff does not push it because it will take time away from private patients." "In this department, there is so much time spent on organization without decision that therapy and supervision time is cut down." "Our department is threatened by the effectiveness of paramedical personnel who meet the needs of the community with these forms of therapy. The department defends its M.D. stronghold by teaching and exposing residents to analytic cases." "We have no such specialists on our staff probably because we are in a rural area." "It seems to be given low priority. The resident picks up cues from his academic environment as to the feelings of his teachers about the relative importance of various topics. Although much lip service is paid to family and conjoint marital therapy and didactic courses may be offered from time to time, no one seems interested in actually doing it, allowing themselves to be watched doing it, or showing others how to do it. If someone is able to do all of the above, he does not seem to get much support from his fellow staff members."

Seventy percent of the residents themselves reported that parapsychiatric personnel seemed much more eager for training in marital and family therapy than were residents in psychiatry.

DISCUSSION

It is obvious that the two authors, who have labored many years in the vineyards of teaching residents the importance of understanding marital and family dynamics and the therapeutic approaches to these problems, espouse the cause of institutionalizing such therapy in the residency training programs. However, we are deeply concerned with the broader problems of residency training and wish to use our surveys to illustrate these problems. Surveys of research training, biological therapy or other areas of psychiatry would, no doubt, uncover similar common difficulties.

The field of psychiatry has become so broad that it is no longer possible to have men for all seasons on the faculty or among the residents. Each has not only his limitations but also individual talents and interests that preclude other areas of expertise. Differences have been discussed in the literature between training for a pluralistic psychiatry as opposed to practicing an eclectic psychiatry. Indeed, there may be a best method for a given patient for which the pluralistic approach would prepare the psychiatrist but unfortunately what usually happens in practice is that the best of the limited number of methods which the given psychiatrist knows is what is used. Resistance to overload and resistance to change are exhibited in faculty and resident alike.

One of our assumptions, that where marital and family therapy training does occur, it is the result of the special interest of one of the faculty members, is borne out by both chairman and resident surveys. This phenomenon fits in with one of the educational goals which is basic to the training of future psychiatrists. It is the fostering of appropriate identification models for the psychiatric resident. Identification is the central mechanism in all programs of education.

As Arlow (8) states: "Organized groups that have an acknowledged history, a continuity of ideology and a body of knowledge to transmit to future generations strive to create a psychological climate that will develop in the students the ideals, the attitudes, and the personal qualities essential for the profession. These goals cannot be achieved by cognitive teaching alone. In any discipline, there is more training than transmission of information. The professional attitude has to be inculcated. An emotional dynamism is required; an identification with leading figures who correspond to the collective ego ideal is the principal instrumentality employed."

Confusion occurs among the residents when appropriate identification models seem at odds with one another and appear to come from different schools of thought. They must decide from evidence presented (if they are fortunate enough to have choices) the adequacy of the articulations of the rationale for the systematic teaching of each of the great variety of therapies. The negative aspects of identification is that the evidence presented does not become the solid basis for conclusions drawn by residents but the identifications themselves may become the decisive factor. Scientific objectivity is lost in the presence of such identifications. Institutionalization of areas of training avoid this danger.

PREDICTIONS OF THE FUTURE

Following Masters and Johnson's (9) report of success in treating sexual problems, psychiatrists have taken a greater interest in treating sexual dysfunction among couples. We feel, and we think this view is shared by most of our colleagues, that the treatment of sexual problems in a couple cannot be separated from the treatment of the relationship between man and woman. If this premise is accurate, to be successful in the treatment of sexual disorders one must also be adept at treating *the couple* with the sexual problem (10). Even the behavioristic methods developed by Masters and Johnson and now under modification in a number of centers across the country involve the couple relationship, and if the sexual difficulties are a consequence rather than a cause of marital disharmony, as we, in our practices, find in 80% of cases, how much more important becomes the acquisition of skills in marital therapy.

Until recently, about the only medical school unit in the country that has been able to provide this training has been the Marriage Council of Philadelphia at the University of Pennsylvania. A few other centers are now developing around the country. As part of this residency program or post-residency training, we recommend at least six months half-time with close supervision, seminars and reading. It seems clear that fortunate circumstances permitted the development of this program at the University of Pennsylvania that will not be possible at many training centers, which may be strong in other areas of psychiatry. To offset such limitations training programs of the future will no longer be able to be provincial. We recommend regional arrangements among psychiatric training institutions such as one now being developed among liberal arts colleges, in a type of consortium. This would permit shifting of residents and faculty from one institution to another. This would decrease the resistances inherent in any local training program to the degree that resistance to innovation can ever be overcome among teachers and students. Some resistance is inevitable. Some is even necessary. But, at least, experimentation and choice of training methods would be greatly encouraged as we take advantage of the pooled resources of the institutions in the consortium. And it would decrease competition for residents and the rapidly diminishing sources of money for training.

REFERENCES

1. Hoch, P. H.: Comments on Graduate Psychiatric Education. *Compr. Psychiatry,* 5:133-136, 1964.
2. Grinker, R. R., Sr.: Psychiatry Rides Madly in All Directions. *Arch. Gen. Psychiatry,* 10:228-237, 1964.
3. Ornstein, P. H.: Sorcerer's Apprentice: The Initial Phase of Training and Education in Psychiatry. *Compr. Psychiatry,* 9:293-315, 1968.
4. Gurin, G., Veroff, J. and Feld, S.: *Americans View Their Mental Health.* New York: Basic Books, 1960.
5. Sager, C. J., et al.: The Married in Treatment. *Arch. Gen. Psychiatry,* 19:205-217, 1968.
6. Group for the Advancement of Psychiatry, Committee on the Family. Integration and Conflict in Family Behavior, Report No. 27, August, 1954.
7. Olson, D. H.: Marital and Family Therapy: Integrated Review and Critique. *J. of Marriage and the Family,* Vol. 32, Nov., 1970, pp. 501-538.
8. Arlow, J. A.: Some Dilemmas in Psychoanalytic Education. *J. Amer. Psychoanalytic Assoc.,* Vol. 20, 556-566, 1972.
9. Masters, W. and Johnson, V.: *Human Sexual Inadequacy.* Boston: Little, Brown and Co., 1970.
10. Lief, H.: "Medical Aspects of Sexuality," in *Cecil-Loeb Textbook of Medicine.* Beeson, Paul B., M.D. and McDermott, Walsh, M.D. (Eds.). Philadelphia: W. B. Saunders Co., pp. 128-131, 1971.

8.

The Psychiatrist's Image of His Role

BERNARD C. HOLLAND, M.D.

and

ROBERT J. STOLLER, M.D.

INTRODUCTION

The thinking behind the decision to spend one day focusing on the education of the psychiatrist was the fact that increasingly psychiatrists are equated with social workers, psychologists, and other allied mental health "emerging" professionals both by the public and the psychiatrists themselves. The question repeatedly arises, is it necessary or wise for the psychiatrist to spend all the time that that he does in his medical training, his internship, and his residency if he is going to end up doing essentially the same thing that others with much less training are said to do equally well. In fact some are wondering if psychiatry is viable as a medical specialty. You can therefore see why the psychiatrist's image of his role is such an important topic for discussion (N. Q. Brill: From a letter planning this meeting).

Few psychiatrists these days can be spared the turmoil that the evolution of our profession has produced. The forces stressing us can be measured at almost every point that defines us as psychiatrists—teaching, research, prevention, methods of treatment, the people to be helped. One cannot seal himself off from these issues.

Nor can we get much comfort by saying these stresses result from the actions of villainous or ignorant people. Each of us knows the legitimacy of the questions raised (even as we question the legitimacy of some of our critics). Issues that led to our present predicament are inherent even in the title of this presentation, for the title implies what does not exist: *the* psychiatrist who has *his* role. In fact, a central issue, which we shall do no more than mention, is: which psychiatrists and which roles? Our image is drawn from the awareness that there are many roles and that these demand many types of psychiatrists. There is no need to list them all, review their functions, or grade their value; besides, the title is only a cover, a calm wording behind which are hidden disturbing problems about the future of psychiatry as a profession, the risks to which it is being subjected, and the question to what extent it serves any but its practitioners.

Our concern over our roles, our value, our usefulness springs from practical issues that are rather new. For the first time, there is hope in our society that psychic pain can be relieved—regardless of the cause, regardless of the diagnosis, regardless of social issues, regardless of moral issues, regardless of the cost. People now believe that, in a democracy attuned to the needs and rights of every citizen, they should not have to suffer their pain. They have been informed (whether accurately or not) that this pain can be relieved safely, that usually the treatment will be mild and minor and will not lead to complications as unseemly as the original symptom. Formerly, those without hope caused no trouble. Having helped bring a steadily increasing hope to society, however, we must pay now, for our optimism has, this far, outrun our armamentarium.

By hard work and with honorable intentions, we created the need, but we have not yet been able to satisfy it*; too many people are hurting. There are not enough psychiatrists, and our methods are too often uncertain, incomplete or insufficient. In addition, much of society's anguish is the result of forces beyond the power of the psychiatrist by himself to prevent, alleviate, or cure. For reasons good and bad, based on realities and on the kinds of fantasies those who claim authority will always attract, attacks have been mounted on our profession—upon our training, body of knowledge, diagnosis, methods of practice, and our commitments (too limited or too unlimited) to society. In our present distress, in the hurt we feel at being misunderstood and having our motives badly judged, we must not forget the bitter core of reality that contributes to our predicament: rising hopes in the midst of unconscionable social inequity and our inability to meet those hopes despite the promise inherent in our healing image. We do not serve ourselves if we only point to the unreasonable forces applied against us: the atmosphere of anti-intellectualism in our society and the turn to magic by those who used to be magically impressed by science; anti-élitism; attacks on the whole medical profession, wherein not only are wrongs perceived as wrong but rights become wrong accusations that, as a profession, our important decisions are guided by greed, provincialism,

* And let us hope we never do, for if all symptoms can be instantly removed, it is the end of society.

stubborn refusal to accept and learn new techniques, and a need to protect a guild.

All medical specialties aim ultimately to achieve their own destruction; that is, the best treatment will be that which is easiest to apply, causes the least immediate disruption, acts rapidly and with full effect, and has no late complications. A treatment that is ideal does not require a trained person, much less a specialist, for its application, as it is completely safe and completely effective. Such a happy outcome, the result of a spread of perfect treatments for the array of disorders a specialty confronts, has yet to strike down any medical specialty, though there are particular signs and symptoms of illness for which this millennium is approaching. As this increasingly happens, all physicians will shift first their practices, then their roles, and finally their identities; nowhere is that more evident than in psychiatry.

Thus we squirm in a pincer, between the increased demand for services (which we psychiatrists cannot yet meet) and the emergence of easily applied, rather safe and simple treatments (such as behavior modification or anxiety-reducing pills) which do not require medical training for their immediate application.* Today, therefore, we must adjust to knowing that we no longer have the image of the strong, intrepid, authoritative, wise healer, kindly in his inability to be of much help, while not yet having reached the day of liberation when treatment will be so complete that we shall no longer be a profession.

THE MEDICAL MODEL

Of course, the medical model. One cannot avoid that discussion; it was inherent in the above.

---

* Though the judgment when they are best used is less simple.

We must look and see: which medical model? The term has been used in several ways. One meaning is that of a belief that emotional disorders are illnesses, with organic etiology; another, of a system of diagnosis either analogous to those of the rest of medicine or coextensive; another, of a style of dealing with patients, from the degree on the stationery, through the white coat, on out to the cost of the treatment; another, the institutional model, that the social agencies concerned—whether federal and state bureaucracies and decision-making bodies, local physical structures like hospitals or storefront clinics, or even the private office of the practitioner—shall be controlled by physicians, with others as ancillaries. Each of these models has been vulnerable to attacks familiar to most of us. These attacks are not without substance; how much one wishes to credit them is a matter of his own prejudices. At any rate, both the attacks and the defenses draw from the above factors regarding the increased demand for care and the new, safer, easily administered types of treatment. Those attacking the medical models say that psychiatry has failed and must forever fail in leading the drive to supply the demand for treatment, that the new treatments do not require skills possessed only by the psychiatrists, and that even those skills do not entitle us to lead treatment programs. The argument against us is not that we should yet cease to be but rather that our usefulness is restricted to a limited number of emotional states.

Albee (1) represents the attack:

> One of the primary arguments used by contemporary psychiatry to support its basic responsibility for the treatment of mental conditions holds that there are underlying organic defects, in most cases still undiscovered, producing the disturbed behavior. Starting from

> this uncertain platform, psychiatry advances the conclusion that medical training, most of which has not been used since the internship, somehow provides unique qualifications to treat these sicknesses.
>
> The gossamer web of logic is not strong enough to hold the weight of this whole proposition, and many contemporary psychiatrists have rejected this argument. In the first place, there is little substantial evidence supporting the hypothesis of an underlying organic defect in most functional mental disorders. Second, the medical training of most psychiatrists was obtained years in the past and is not especially relevant to their therapeutic activities. In other situations, where the stakes are different, most psychiatrists have refused to practice medicine in any traditional sense . . .
>
> Third, when a real organic cause is discovered to be the significant underlying factor in the production of disturbed behavior (as has been the case in a few genuine mental diseases), then the treatment of these conditions is removed from the psychiatric field.

Not bad, and certainly not an extremist position.

Especially in regard to a medical model for the etiologies of psychic disorders, many of us would agree with Albee that it has its limitations. We believe with him that many states of psychic pain, while needing a biological substrate for their existence, are the result of environmental stresses, such as interpersonal relationships. Additionally, we believe that the biological changes resultant from these stresses are often not comparable to those we call physical disease, such as, say, delirium tremens. Few would deny that a medical model for etiology (in the above sense) is inappropriate for most of the pain and unhappiness of humanity. Many of us would also agree that we do not have a monopoly on the treatment of many of these "non-medical" disorders. Therapists, from psychoanalysts to strict behaviorists, have proven their worth without a medical degree.

Let us suggest, instead, that the medical model to be considered not be that for etiologies or diagnostic systems but rather that to which the title of our presentation attends: our role, even more, our identity. It will be hard for our critics to argue that the identity of *physician,* even with all its variations among the specialties, is the same as that of other professions.* So let us look into that identity to find other medical models more worth our concern. The first we can note is built upon the sense of responsibility. This, inculcated in the physician when he is a student, intern, and resident, never to be relinquished, is not comparable to that found in any other profession (though the personality qualities of others may be as laudable as those of the best physicians). In fact, there is a need in those people who choose to become physicians to fix that intense sense of responsibility as part of their identity. It results from a long tradition and it burns itself into one's soul. The tradition, for those self-selected to serve it, is a model, carried unendingly inside, on which to base identity and behavior. It is no meager model; the need to approximate it so dominates us that the failure to live up to its impossible demands is probably the primary reason that the suicide rate is so high among physicians and highest among psychiatrists.

A second medical model, inculcated into us from the beginning, is the concept of dynamics, in most medicine represented by physiology and, in regard to psychic function, by neurophysiology and psychodynamics. We are committed to

* And to point to the failure of some physicians to develop and live by that identity is no argument against the thesis, only against the failure of these physicians.

the scientific-philosophic position that the mechanisms that underlie and lead to a sign or symptom, a syndrome or disease, ought to be understood. In a selfish sense, the search for this understanding makes the physician's practice exciting and gratifying; more important, it increases the chances he will do the best job of determining what is wrong so that the best possible treatment can be applied; in the largest sense, such curiosity is a basis of research into causes and treatments. In psychiatry, especially under the influence of non-medical experts (e.g. behavior therapists), an attitude is growing that such understanding and the desire to understand even more is unnecessary. This belief extends even into those political bodies that, disguised as scientific institutions, direct the future of psychiatry by the manner they grant funds.

Yet understanding of dynamics is *not* necessary for much of the treatment done by the general psychiatrist in his day-to-day work. Perhaps this attitude is most outspoken among those practicing behavior modification or EST, who when able in fact to modify behavior or mood to a more comfortable state, can show empirically that an understanding of etiology or psychodynamics was not necessary to relieve their patients' distress. But that perspective is like strip-mining; it destroys the future to feed the present. Were it to possess everyone, further knowledge of the "physiology" of human behavior would be precipitously slowed (until, in panic, we restored the dynamic model).

We wish to return again to the diagnosis model, which, seen in a different light, we offer as a third medical model invaluable for our society. Herein, the term "medical" does not need to suggest that these conditions are purely biological or identical in their formation with the classically "medical" diseases. Yet the concept of diagnosis, an essential theme only for physicians, can raise the quality of treatment, research, and conceptualization in psychic disorders. We would suggest the following model. A diagnosis is arrived at in the rest of medicine when one has first delineated a syndrome (a collection of signs and symptoms) underlying which are pathophysiological mechanisms whose surface manifestations are the signs and symptoms of the syndrome; at bottom are the etiological factors, which in each case are the same and cause the pathophysiology that surfaces as the syndrome. That medical model for diagnosis is possible in psychiatric diagnoses as well. Unfortunately, our problems are complex, and so, in regard to many conditions, we are still at the first stage (through which the rest of medicine passed a half century or more ago), that of defining syndromes. Having done so, we shall still, in the future, have to delineate the dynamics. (In the psychiatric disorders that are truly diseases, these will be found in pathophysiology, as in the rest of medicine, but in the greatest part of what now concerns the psychiatrist, the dynamics will be psychodynamics, without physiological implications.) Then, in some exciting era to come, we shall also know the multidetermined factors that set the pathological dynamic processes in motion.

That is a model; it is the one created from and within medicine, and it is shared by no other profession. We give it up at the greatest risk.

Our fourth medical model, like the others, is, especially, an attitude, and therefore becomes, in the best circumstances, a piece of identity. It is the philosophic position, inculcated invariably and unendingly throughout one's medical training and subsequent career, that the human is, in all his humanity, also a biological organism. That is not a notion one paints on his surface from a bit of reading and an inspirational lecture or two. One immerses his hands in it in the anatomy and physiology lab; he absorbs it from biochemists and histologists, from molecular biologists and statisticians; he reinforces it as he does physical examinations and surgical procedures; it is driven into him by all the mechanisms of learning, by the power of his fantasy life, and by the insatiable hunger that the learning process in medicine creates. It does not get there by magic; he must study it and absorb it by living it. It cannot come easily, and it cannot come without knowledge. It cannot come by faith alone; it is not served by lip service.

And it is in even those of us who move so far from our past that we never again enter an operating room, or read an x-ray, or do a physical examination. In our psychotherapeutic or analytic work, we still sense our patients' physiology; it serves to alert us to somatic factors that masquerade as physical. But, even more, it is there as a dimension to our institution—to the play of our unconscious with the patient's—that cannot exist in the non-physician. With it, we may sense dim, primeval movements stirring in our patients the sounds of which no other instrument can catch.

APPREHENSIONS

Even if our profession does not, in all its individual members, live up to what it best can do and stand for, even if the needs are greater than what at present we can satisfy, and even if many treatments are now safe enough that those applying them do not need the cautions and skills that medical education provides, society had better not dispense yet with the medical model. Certainly there can be shifting of priorities, and hopefully many aspects of treatment can be taken over by non-physicians. In some cases, adept non-physicians may have available to them techniques of treatment that they can apply better than anyone else (certain lay psychoanalysts are an obvious example). But if society wishes to be rid of the above four models—if it is felt that the people who will take on the responsibility of patient care will function perfectly well without such qualities built into their identity and reflected in their roles—then the future, up until the time when all treatments are safe and uncomplicated, will be a dangerous one for many of the emotionally disabled.

And who in the future—which profession when acting at the height of its powers—will praise, love, encourage, and practice researches that reach from cell function to dreaming, from the infant to his society, from the brain to the mind? Who will seek out responsibility to take the discoveries still to come in the neurosciences, endocrinology, genetics, and the like and those from such as psychoanalysis, behaviorism, and ethology and interweave these into the treatment of the particular patient and into the effort to prevent emotional or social disorder?

In these days of the relevant, and in the rush to earlier specialization, we find that medical educators and their students are covertly agreeing with our critics. Certainly, the right to proper care for all of our citizens cannot be met without more efficient and effective treatments, better distribution of care, and, perhaps, more practitioners. Of course, more practitioners who can alleviate pain, whether they are physicians or not, will be a relief (as long as all practice safely).

In fact, if the issue is simply one of delivery of services, then our modern medical educators are cheating on their own principles. Why not really plunge in and speed up the process of education even more in order to meet the goal of more therapists. If the medical model is such an encumbrance, just cut out the first two years of medical school entirely. That, plus removing the internship and streamlining residencies with tracks, would create practitioners much more quickly and leave them unhindered by the esoterica of science. We could develop large numbers of people competent to administer antibiotics, EST, behavioral modification, hormones, or take out appendices, tonsils and gall bladders—and none would have to have experienced the basic sciences of medicine. The quality of the practice would probably not be inferior to that done by the average physician in America today. And we should make every effort to create large numbers of such midwives and battalion surgeons. The skills they develop will be more dependable in their hands than if most of us tried to do the same things. Society needs that help; we should encourage it.

But who will take care of the emergency when the applied treatment goes wrong; who will comprehend the complications? Who will know the underlying physiology and psychodynamics; who will ask the questions that evolve into the experiments needed for tomorrow's knowledge? Who will know how to abstract from the concrete problem to today in order to create the future?

Grinker (2) says:

> In understanding an unhappy, ineffective individual who is seeking help, systems of communication, understanding, and then interpretation—or suportive, educational, or directive techniques—are appropriately utilized. With full sanction these are employed in varying

> depths or degrees of intensity by middle-aged housewives, pastors, nurses, social workers, and psychologists, as well as by pychiatrists. It is therefore clear that of all therapies psychotherapy is the least medical. The problem rests on the fact that the persons enumerated above utilize, with varying degrees of skill, the same general method of treatment for all conditions.
>
> The truly medical model is one in which psychotherapy is only a part. The total field in terms of therapy includes differential diagnosis involving considerations of organic brain disease and other somatic afflictions; diagnosis of specific nosological categories about which something of the natural history and prognosis is known; the choice of therapeutic environment, such as home, clinic, or hospital; the choice of therapy such as drugs, shock, and psychotherapy; orientation toward individuals, groups, and family; and such choices as behavioral therapy, or psychoanalysis, etc.
>
> Indeed, psychiatry as a whole constitutes an expanded field that can be envisioned best as a system without sacrificing any of its parts.

That is an important point; it is "thc total field"—the interrelating energies and capabilities that "system" implies—that no other profession can bring to our present problems of the delivery of proper health care, the improvement of treatment, and the advancement of knowledge in research. We must not lose sight, because of the emerging demands in our society for decent treatment, of the issues raised by the concepts of "field" or "system."

While significant, we do not feel that the argument is properly focused when proponents of one system or another of treatment point up to the inadequacies of others and the superiority of their own. Most techniques of treatment are easily learned by anyone, and until the beautiful day of the future, the treatments used today in psychiatry are often only partly effective. Nonetheless, the day will come when the psychiatrist will no longer have a role distinct enough to warrant his present eminence in decision-making. That day will come when the perfect treatments are developed. Before that, we should expect the psychiatrist to lose his importance only when other professions develop members who are biologists of the human animal, broadly trained in the many perspectives of the psychology of humans, skillful in diagnosis and evaluation of best treatments to be used, and trustworthy in the sense of responsibility comparable to that traditional for the physician. The other professions need be no more than that.

Of course, nowadays, such a person is called a psychiatrist.

REFERENCES

1. Albee, George W.: Emerging Concepts of Mental Illness and Models of Treatment: The Psychological Point of View. *Amer. J. Psychiat.*, 125: 870-876, 1969.
2. Grinker, Roy R., Sr.: Emerging Concepts of Mental Illness and Models of Treatment: The Medical Point of View. *Amer. J. Psychiat.*, 125: 865-869, 1969.

9.

The Education of Tomorrow's Psychiatrists

PETER F. REGAN, M.D.

and

S. MOUCHLY SMALL, M.D.

Our crystal ball has become clouded so we can only see the barest outlines of the future of medical education. To compound our predictive dilemmas, these ghost-like forms appear to change at an accelerating pace. Social changes involving the entire organization of medical care, rapidly changing educational strategies and a reconceptualization of the profession of medicine and what constitutes illness have all contributed to a feeling of instability. Thus, especially in the field of psychiatry we are deeply aware of the need for a sense of direction.

Fortunately, we can begin our planning with assurance that *all* will not be new. We can start from a reasonably firm base: our concept of the essential characteristics of a psychiatrist as formulated by Drs. Holland and Stoller (1). In this concept the psychiatrist has comprehensive knowledge and understanding of the physical and behavioral dynamics of the human being, possesses diagnostic skill and therapeutic judgment, and operates within the professional code of medical ethics coupled with a deep sense of responsibility. An additional criterion of a profession is its self-governance and self-regulation which are intended to guarantee the continuing competence of its members for the protection of its clients or patients (2). This, too, must be incorporated in any educational program.

These enduring characteristics and responsibilities of the psychiatrist provide the basic framework for designing his educational plan. But the psychiatrist has to be prepared to practice intelligently and efficiently in the society of the 1980s and 1990s and longer. Our educational program must prepare him to meet current demands and provide the groundwork for future practice in conjunction with an orientation toward continuing education and lifelong habits of scholarship. Before outlining a suggested educational model, let us take a brief glance at the background . . . at the changes now underway in our society, in health care and in medical education.

THE DIRECTIONS OF CHANGE

It is relatively easy to see some of the changes that will have an ever increasing impact on psychiatry and psychiatric education. As the United States and other developed nations move into a post-industrial society, one of the most pervasive of these changes is an apparently inexorable expansion of the demand for services. This increasing demand is both quantitative and qualitative. There is a demand for more creature comforts, and for more public services like health care, education, social welfare, comunications and transportation. But there is also a demand that these services be improved, that they be distributed more equitably and that they be under continual consumer surveillance.

The whole field of health care, including psychiatry, is caught up in this movement. Between 1955 and 1970, for example, the number of people employed in the United States health care system increased from 2.5 to 4.0 million and the national expenditures for health rose from 4.7% (approximately $17.9 billion) to 7.1% of the Gross National Product [GNP] (approximately $67.2 billion) (3). The number of psychiatrists in the U.S. has doubled in each of the last three decades. Hand in hand with expansion has gone specialization. There are now more than 125 health professions and occupations (with 375 titles listed within the health services industry) (4). As in other service fields, growth has been accompanied by increased governmental support: governmental expenditures for health comprised 23.4% of the national total expenditures in 1955, 39.9% in 1970.

It is obvious that this rate of expansion cannot continue forever, and there is already much public furor aimed at controlling the rising expenditures for health. But the eventual limits on the size and course of the health care system are on a collision course with ever-mounting public demands. Health care has been accepted as a universal right, and we now hear constant calls for improvement and extension: for faster, better and more personalized treatment of acute illnesses; for vast improvement in the care of the chronically ill and aged; for new advances in prevention and for the enhancement of health; and for effective action on problems which the health professions cannot handle alone, such as alcoholism and drug addiction.

What are the developing answers to these trends? For the health care system, the major trends include: some form of universal health insurance; regionalized systems of care, with increasing control mechanisms to assure adequate access and coverage to all citizens; a relative stability in the doctor-population ratio, but an increase in the number of people working in the other health professions and occupations; more utilization of health care teams, with delegation of more medical responsibilities to others; interdisciplinary efforts related to prevention, chronic illness, aging, and socio-medical problems, with the health professions serving in an auxiliary rather than a central capacity; increasing pressure for quality control by periodic relicensure and re-certification (5).

On the educational side, several responses can be observed. These include: abbreviated formal education with earlier specialization encouraged by multiple-track systems; a relative de-emphasis of basic research in natural sciences accompanied by growing emphasis on teaching for service and on social research; periodic and systematic cycles of continuing education throughout the professional's life (6); direct involvement of the educational enterprise in the realities of health care (by a variety of mechanisms including taking responsibility for health maintenance programs, providing education in community resources rather than in university hospitals, etc.); the imposition of controls on completely free choice of specialty (by restricting opportunities in such fields as surgery, while expanding opportunity in such fields as family practice) and increasing curricular emphasis on preparation for team work by interdisciplinary programs with a heavy social science base.

This has been a cursory review of the forces of change

in health care and medical education. Admittedly, each reader can add to the list, and certainly all of us are aware of larger issues looming in the background: the demand for equality, the energy crisis, the environmental problem. The review, however, does make our educational problem clear. We must in some fashion design a program which will be congruent with the overall patterns of health education and of health care ... and both of these patterns are in a state of dramatic flux.

NEW DIMENSIONS IN PSYCHIATRIC EDUCATION

Confronted with this problem, we must be prepared to make drastic modifiations in our present educational methods in psychiatry. We must view psychiatric education as a lifelong continuum, we must reach a better appraisal of what is essential and what is elective in that educational pattern, and we must orient our thinking to educational objectives rather than to blocks of time.

Psychiatric Education as a Lifelong Continuum

We have long since passed the period when it was reasonable to look at medical education and psychiatric education as a sort of layer cake, progressing in lock step fashion from undergraduate education to basic sciences to clinical work in medical school through internship to residency and eventuating in a "finished product." The days of uniformity are gone; there are enormous variations and discrepancies among entering medical students, among the programs of different medical schools, and among tracks in the same school. This diversity and the speed of medical advances and of societal changes make the concept of a "finished product" an absurdity.

In this real situation, we cannot much longer adhere to such notions as a three-year residency in psychiatry. The present preparation of students is so variable that three years may be too much for some and too little for others. Long or short though it may be, it is not final; it must be continually renewed by systematic continuing education.

Appraisal of the Essential and the Elective

A single evening spent with modern psychiatric literature will serve to convince us that we cannot embrace all knowledge in the whole field. Contributions are made by disciplines ranging from biophysics to ethology, and involve psychiatric subspecializations of all sorts: child psychiatry, community psychiatry, forensic psychiatry, administrative psychiatry and the various therapeutic subspecialties like family therapy, behavior therapy, etc. It is impossible to incorporate all of this diversity into a single educational sequence. Even if it were possible it would be unwise, *for what is desired is variation built on a common base, not uniformity.*

We must return, therefore, to the basic characteristics of the psychiatrist—knowledge of the biological and behavioral dynamics, diagnostic skill and therapeutic judgment and professional ethics. These must constitute the core of an educational program from which elective opportunities in other disciplines and in the subspecialties of psychiatry may spring.

An Orientation to Educational Objectives

To orient ourselves to these characteristics of psychiatrists is to orient ourselves toward educational objectives rather than to time spent in school or residency training. We must come to some agreement about the level of knowledge and skill the psychiatrist must possess and then design and use evaluation instruments to determine if he has reached the necessary level (and, later, to determine if he is maintaining the necessary level) (7). Fortunately, our capacities for evaluation are improving. While still cumbersome and inadequate insofar as measuring clinical competence is concerned, they are rapidly improving, and research should give us adequate tools within the next few years (8).

A LIFELONG EDUCATIONAL SEQUENCE

With these educational dimensions it seems possible to design an education sequence in psychiatry that preserves the essential characteristics of the psychiatrist, provides opportunities for flexibility, and is amenable to shifts in education and health care. Such a sequence is presented here with a plea for understanding; it is presented without apology, but equally without dogmatism; it is presented with an awareness of its crudeness and limitations, in the hope that examination of it may lead to real improvement in our present system.

Substantially, this sequence involves five phases of psychiatric education.

I—Basic Medical Education
II—Basic Psychiatric Education
III—Advanced Psychiatric Education
IV—Elective Psychiatric Education
V—Systematic Continuing Education

The estimated time necessary for completion of each phase is indicated only for purposes of general orientation, and it must be understood that completion of the phase would be determined by evaluative procedures rather than simple duration of time.

PHASE I—BASIC MEDICAL EDUCATION

Educational Objectives:

1. Acquisition of basic understanding of the human being biologically and behaviorally, in illness and in health, in the context of his society and culture.
2. Acquisition of basic skills in the diagnosis and treatment of common physical illnesses.
3. Learning and observance of medical codes of ethics and attitudes of professionalism toward one's work.

Teaching Methods: This phase would normally be completed in undergraduate and medical school work. It would involve learning experiences in laboratories and in a variety of general medical situations in which the psychiatric faculty would also participate. Close working relationships with respected clinicians would foster identification and the assimilation of medical ethics. If these elements are not provided in medical school (and some multiple track plans may indeed fall short in this respect), special provisions must be made for compensatory work at the beginning of specialty training. Already, it is sometimes necessary to "round out" the preparation of a beginning psychiatric resident with some assignments to Medicine or to the Emergency Room.

Evaluation Procedure: Objective testing (including improved versions of patient management problems and other clinical evaluative methodologies), and evaluation by faculty, fellow students, and patients.

PHASE II—BASIC PSYCHIATRIC EDUCATION

Educational Objectives:

1. Acquisition of basic knowledge and skills in the diagnosis of major and common psychiatric conditions.
2. The development of rudimentary skills in psychiatric treatment and management.
3. Acquisition of a minimum cursory familiarity with major explanations of behavior and psychiatric illness, including biological, social, psychological, and psychoanalytic schools.

Teaching Methods: The student should have individual responsibility for diagnosis and treatment of at least three patients with each major illness category, probably requiring experience both inside and outside a hospital, under close supervision by psychiatric faculty. Engagement in team efforts or subspecialty activities should be held to a minimum until this basic competence is acquired.

Timing of Learning Opportunity: Developing multiple-track systems will allow many students to complete this introductory phase while still in medical school; for others, it will constitute the first portion of residency training. At either level, it would seem that the educational objectives could be achieved with six months of full-time effort or its equivalent.

Evaluation Procedure: Objective testing of cognitive skills and clinical competence stressing communicative skills, patient-doctor relationship and professional attitudes through faculty evaluations.

PHASE III—ADVANCED PSYCHIATRIC EDUCATION

Educational Objectives:

1. Acquisition of advanced skills in history taking, psychiatric examination and diagnosis.
2. Competence in the selection and application of major treatment methodologies.
3. Development of basic competency in group management.
4. Acquisition of basic knowledge and skills in chosen subspecialty areas.
5. Design and initiation of research projects.

Teaching Methods: Rotation through a variety of clinical situations with assured participation in child psychiatry, forensic psychiatry, neurology, community psychiatry, consultation services, ward management, and group/family therapy. Faculty should be drawn from related fields as well as from departments of psychiatry.

Timing of Learning Opportunity: A few students will have entered this phase in medical school. For most, it will be entirely experienced during specialty training. It is estimated that the educational objectives can be achieved within an 18-month period of full-time effort.

Evaluation Procedure:

1. Objective testing as indicated above.
2. Faculty supervision and evaluation of work with patients.
3. Initiation of an approved research project.

PHASE IV—ELECTIVE PSYCHIATRIC EDUCATION

Educational Objectives:

1. Acquisition of advanced knowledge and skill in a selected area of psychiatry.
2. Completion of research project.

Teaching Methods: Clearly, these will vary according to the field which the student may choose. The work may be oriented toward basic science or clinical activity, and may be concentrated in any subspecialty area of psychiatry.

Timing of Learning Opportunity: This flexible phase of education may last months or years, depending on the field of activity.

Evaluation Procedure:

1. Highly specialized techniques will have to be used according to the field of choice.
2. Completion of research project.

PHASE V—SYSTEMATIC CONTINUING EDUCATION

Educational Objectives:

1. Maintenance and up-dating of skills and knowledge in the face of scientific and social change.

Educational Methods: Nationally coordinated programs involving 400-500 hours of learning in every five-year period.

Evaluation Procedure: Expanded and refined national testing procedures along the lines of developing self-assessment tests, with stress on patient-management problems and clinical competence.

DISCUSSION

In this brief outline of a suggested sequence many details are omitted. For example, it is our personal view that the education of a psychiatrist must involve active work and participation in settings ranging from community walk-in clinics to State Hospitals. Such elements, however, are blueprint details... and we have attempted to maintain our focus on overall directions.

Clearly, the directions suggested by the authors carry a certain cost, principally one of conceptualization. We will have to forego two cherished images: that of "*The* Psychiatrist" and that of "*The* Psychiatric Residency." These monolithic concepts are already at variance with the reality of highly diverse working patterns in Psychiatry and the equal diversity of educational programs. But they still remain abstract goals, placing the impossible burden of universality on student and educator alike, while simultaneously locking the student and the educator into an inflexible and unrealistic time-frame.

The benefits of surrendering these absolutist concepts are impressive: flexibility of time, flexibility of location, flexibility of career. Consider the options for a student at various phases of his educational program:

> At the medical school level, he may concentrate on the fundamentals of psychiatry, confident that his efforts will shorten his later educational time sequence; conversely, he may delve deeply into basic science, confident that the basic elements of psychiatry will be available later.
>
> For special training at the advanced level, he may enter a training program with assurance (a) that it will provide him with a general competence, (b) that the speed of his progress will be determined by his ability and not by a fixed time period, and (c) that as his experience indicates which subspecialty area he wishes to pursue, he will have access to it by transferring to another program if it is not available at his own place of training.
>
> At each juncture, he will be assured that continued, individualized opportunities for more depth and more breadth will be available, guided by self-assessment through continuing education programs. He will not be trapped in the present "now or never" dilemma.

As a rule, educational flexibility of this sort imposes extra burdens on the educator. In the present proposal, however, gains would seem to outweigh losses. Admittedly, educators will be challenged to develop more adequate methods of assessment and evaluation at different levels of education.

This is difficult, and will require a redirection of effort toward areas like educational technology, testing techniques, and curricular development with which most of us are too unfamiliar.

Such a redirection of effort seems inevitable in any case, however. Even if our consciences (our "professional ethics" as educators, if you will) would allow us to persist in defining the educational program in terms of three years, the public will not long allow us to do so.

Without in any way minimizing these difficulties, or the logistic problems involved, it must be recognized that the educator will share emancipation with the student:

> The Department Chairman will no longer be obliged to encompass every element of mental health in a department with a limited number of positions. He will be able to concentrate on the basics and on selected subspecialties, knowing that students desirous of other subspecialties will have options for transfer.
>
> The faculty as a whole will no longer have to indulge in the fantasy of an encyclopedic curriculum; the curriculum will not be the end, but the beginning, of the student's lifelong learning.
>
> The faculty will be able to stop once and for all the paradox that now imposes itself each spring, as a group of third-year residents approach their thirty-sixth month and each one differs from his peers. "Completion" of a phase of education may come at any time (shorter or longer than the time spans suggested above, as the case may be). It will come by achievement and evaluation, however, and not by the magic of a turned page on a calendar.

There will be those who will attack these suggestions as compounding an administrative nightmare—involving problems of funding, responsibility for longitudinal records of each individual, transferability of credits among many others. Perhaps regionalization of educational and training efforts may help to overcome some of these valid concerns.

However, we see a multi-level, phased program as one which will allow us to break out of the shackles of time and space. It allows for designing and operating a sequential program in a number of locations—a student could conceivably take each of the five phases in a different locus rather than being locked into a single "residency program"—and different students would proceed at different paces. Indeed, the future may well see many elements even more decentralized, as we discover how properly to utilize mass media, programmed instruction, etc., but that is material for another paper.

In summary, we have attempted to present an approach to teaching tomorrow's psychiatrists. It is an approach which will require readjustments, a lifelong orientation, with phases of instruction being linked to educational achievement and evaluation rather than to lapsed time, and with maximum opportunity for diversity and subspecialization. Some such plan is necessary if we are to respond adequately to the shifting worlds of education and health care, while also preserving the basic elements of our profession.

REFERENCES

1. Holland, B. C. and Stoller, R. J.: The Psychiatrist's Image of His Role, in this volume, p. 151.
2. Friedson, E.: *Profession of Medicine.* New York: Dodd, Mead & Co., 1971, pp. 71-84.
2. U.S. Dept. of Health, Education & Welfare: *Towards a Comprehensive Health Policy for the 1970's—A White Paper.* Washington, D. C.: U.S. Govt. Printing Office, May 1971, pp. 19-21.

4. U.S. Dept. of Health, Education & Welfare: Public Health Service Publication No. 263, Sec. 21. Washington, D. C.: U.S. Govt. Printing Office, 1970.
5. Carmichael, H. T., Small, S. M., and Regan, P. F.: *Prospects and Proposals: Lifetime Learning for Psychiatrists.* Washington, D.C.: American Psychiatric Association, 1972.
6. Regan, P. F. and Small, S. M.: Toward a Continuum of Formal and Continuing Education. *Amer. J. Psychiatry,* 128:607-609, 1971.
7. Small, S. M.: Self-Renewal: The Theme of the Seventies. *Amer. J. Psychiatry,* 128:124-126, 1972.
8. Small, S. M. and Regan, P. F.: An Evaluation of Evaluations. Presented at Annual Meeting of the American Psychiatric Association, Hawaii, May, 1973.